C0-APY-059

Boehringer Ingelheim

**Boehringer Ingelheim
Pharmaceuticals, Inc.**
a subsidiary of
Boehringer Ingelheim Corporation
90 East Ridge
P.O. Box 368
Ridgefield, Connecticut 06877

A Valuable Addition to Your Medical Library...

Dear Doctor:

Boehringer Ingelheim Pharmaceuticals, Inc. is proud to bring you this updated second edition of HEMATOLOGY FOR THE HOUSE OFFICER by Larry Waterbury, M.D.

This useful volume will assist you in the diagnosis and treatment of hematologic disorders. It focuses on problems facing the clinician and outlines logical steps to solving these problems. This second edition has been completely revised and the references updated. New sections have been added on fibrinolytic therapy and platelet dysfunction.

We hope you find this manual a valuable addition to your medical library.

Sincerely,

Penelope A. Bowers, M.D.
Associate Director, Clinical Investigation

PAB:ab

Telephone: (203)438-0311
Telex: 221091 Answer back BI PHARMA

Hematology for the House Officer

SECOND EDITION

Larry Waterbury, M.D.

Head, Hematology and Medical Oncology Division
Baltimore City Hospitals
Associate Professor of Medicine
Johns Hopkins University School of Medicine
Baltimore, Maryland

WILLIAMS & WILKINS
Baltimore/London

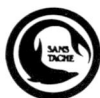

Editor: James L. Sangston
Associate Editor: Jonathan W. Pine, Jr.
Design: JoAnne Janowiak
Illustration Planning: Joseph P. Cummings
Production: Carol Eckhart

Copyright © 1984
Williams & Wilkins
428 East Preston Street
Baltimore, MD 21202, U.S.A.

All rights reserved. This book is protected by copyright. No part of this book may be reproduced in any form or by any means, including photocopying, or utilized by any information storage and retrieval system without written permission from the copyright owner.

Accurate indications, adverse reactions, and dosage schedules for drugs are provided in this book, but it is possible that they may change. The reader is urged to review the package information data of the manufacturers of the medications mentioned.

Made in the United States of America

First Edition, 1980
 Reprinted 1981, 1982, 1983

Library of Congress Cataloging in Publication Data

Main entry under title:

Waterbury, Larry.
 Hematology for the house officer.

 Includes index.
 1. Blood—Diseases—Handbooks, manuals, etc. 2. Hematology—Handbooks, mauals, etc. I. Title. [DNLM: 1. Hematology—Handbooks. WH 39 W324h]
 RC636.W33 1984   616.1'5   84-2181
 ISBN 0-683-08852-1

86 87 88 89   10 9 8 7 6 5 4 3 2

Dedication

To my wife Marcia

Preface

As with the first edition, the purpose of this second edition of <u>Hematology for the House Officer</u> is to assist house officers in the diagnosis and treatment of hematologic disorders. It continues to focus on problems as they present to the clinician and to attempt to outline logical steps to problem solving. All sections have been revised and references updated. New sections have been added on fibrinolytic therapy and platelet dysfunction.

I am gratified by the popularity of the first edition of this manual and hope this second edition will continue to meet a need for the busy house officer dealing with clinical problems.

Acknowledgments

ACKNOWLEDGMENTS

This manual was reviewed by a number of house officers at Baltimore City Hospitals, and I am grateful to them for their comments and suggestions. In particular I would like to thank Doctors Adam Blacksin, Ben Jones, Larry Appel, Lloyd Stahl, Rich Josephson, Mary Korytkowski, Bill Russell and Bob Weisgrau. I am very appreciative of the excellent professional clerical efforts of Mrs. Carole Messman.

About The Author

ABOUT THE AUTHOR

Larry Waterbury, M.D. is head of the Division of Hematology and Oncology at Baltimore City Hospitals, and Associate Professor of Medicine at the Johns Hopkins University School of Medicine. He was formerly an Instructor in Medicine at Southwestern Medical School in Dallas, Texas, where he did his residency in internal medicine and fellowship in hematology and oncology.

Contents

Chapter 1

Anemia: Introduction and Approach to Diagnosis

ANEMIA: GENERAL CONSIDERATIONS

Normal hematocrit (Hct) and hemoglobin (Hgb) levels vary among laboratories and methods of determination. However, in general, anemia is present in adults when the Hct is reproducibly less than 42% in men or 37% in women or when the Hgb level is less than 14 g% in men or 12 g% in women. A number of in vivo and in vitro variables affect

Table 1.1
Hematocrit Variations Throughout Life

	Hct
Term newborn (cord blood)	44-62
Term newborn (capillary blood)	53-68
Infant (3 months)	30-38
Child (10 years)	37-44
Pregnancy (30 weeks gestation)	26-34
Adult female	37-47
Adult male	42-54

these values and must be taken into consideration. Every house officer at some time encounters a puzzling Hct change in a newly admitted patient between the value obtained in the emergency room and the value obtained on the floor a few hours or a day later. Rather than bleeding or hemolysis, one or more of the following variables are usually to blame and are assessed by asking the following questions:

What is the state of the patient's hydration?

- Hct swings as high as 6-8% may occur with correction of dehydration or volume overload.

How was the blood specimen obtained?

- Hgb/Hct values are frequently higher from a fingerstick

1

(heel stick, earlobe) than from a venous sample unless excessive pressure is applied to facilitate blood flow (lowers the hematocrit).

- Prolonged stasis from a tourniquet increases the hematocrit, as do muscular activity and cold.

- Hct drops of several points may be seen between samples taken from a patient who is sitting and those taken after the patient has been lying down a few minutes (increases in plasma volume when supine).

Table 1.2
Variables Which Tend to Raise the Hematocrit

Dehydration
Fingerstick (heelstick, earlobe) samples
Prolonged tourniquet stasis
Exposure to cold
Increased muscular activity
Upright position
Centrifugation techniques (especially with bizarre cell shapes)

Variables Which Tend to Decrease the Hematocrit

Volume overload
Supine position
Capillary tube leakage during centrifugation
Automated techniques

How was the Hct/Hgb determined?

If manual method, remember:

- Capillary tube Hcts are very reproducible (1-2% variability only). Manual hemoglobin methods are less accurate.

- Microhematocrits are frequently slightly higher than automated hematocrits (see below) because of plasma trapping (this is increased when red cells are misshapen, as in sickle cell disease and severe iron deficiency).

- Watch out for an occult leak from the poorly sealed capillary Hct tube.

If an automated method is used:

Most laboratories now use automated methods for the complete blood count (CBC). Routine data obtained usually include the Hct, Hgb, red cell count (RBC) mean corpuscular volume (MCV), mean corpuscular hemoglobin (MCH) and mean corpuscular hemoglobin concentration (MCHC). The following equations describe the relationships between these data:

$$MCV = Hct \div RBC \text{ (in cubic micrometers, or femtoliters, fl)}$$
$$MCH = Hgb \div RBC \text{ (in picograms, pg)}$$
$$MCHC = Hgb \div Hct \text{ (in grams/100 ml RBCs, g/dl RBCs)}$$

One commonly used automated system (Coulter) measures directly the Hgb, RBC and MCV and from these measured variables calculates the Hct, MCH and MCHC. In another system (SMA) the RBC and the Hgb are measured directly and the hematocrit is estimated from a measure of whole blood conductivity (MCV, MCH and MCHC are calculated). The major advantage of the automated system — other than the obvious advantages of speed, automated printout, etc. — is a high degree of reproducibility. The indices, especially the MCV, are precise values which can reliably be used in approaching the diagnostic workup of anemia.

The MCV is a measure of cell size and is more reproducible than one's ability to tell subtle changes in size from the examination of the peripheral smear. The MCH is a measure of the average amount of hemoglobin in each individual cell (essentially giving the same information as the MCV). The MCHC is a measure of the concentration of hemoglobin in each cell (a measure of chromicity).

Table 1.3
Representative Normal Values (Coulter S)

	Adult Male	Adult Female
Hgb (g/dl blood)	14–18	12–16
Hct (%)	42–54	37–47
MCV (fl)	82–98	82–98
MCH (pg)	27–32	27–32
MCHC (g/dl RBCs)	31.5–36	31.5–36

HELP FROM THE PERIPHERAL SMEAR:

The peripheral smear may give helpful and sometimes even definitive diagnostic information in the evaluation of anemia. Except at the extremes of cell size, the electronically measured MCV is superior

to the peripheral smear in determining RBC size. However, RBC shape,
chromicity, inclusions, etc. have definite diagnostic importance.
Table 1.4 lists common conditions associated with various RBC morphologies.

Table 1.4
Common Causes of Various RBC Abnormalities

Hypochromia, Microcytosis:	Iron deficiency Thalassemia Sideroblastic anemia Chronic inflammation
Macrocytosis:	Liver disease (central targeting) Megaloblastic anemia (macroovalocytes) Reticulocytosis Newborn Preleukemia (mimics megaloblastic morphology)
Marked Anisocytosis and Poikilocytosis:	Marked iron deficiency Megaloblastic anemia (severe) Microangiopathic hemolysis Leukoerythroblastosis Hemoglobinopathies
Target Cells:	Liver disease C hemoglobin (AC, CC, SC) SS disease Postsplenectomy Thalassemia Artifact
Spiculated RBCs:	Hereditary acanthocytosis Liver disease (spur cells) Renal disease (burr cells) Post splenectomy Hypothyroidism Microangiopathic hemolysis
Tear Drop Cells:	Leukoerythroblastosis Megaloblastic anemias Thalassemia
Howell-Jolly Bodies:	Postsplenectomy Megaloblastic Anemia Erythroleukemia

(Continued on following page)

Table 1.4 Cont'd

Pappenheimer Bodies:	Postsplenectomy Sideroblastic anemia Megaloblastic anemia Alcohol Marked hemolysis Thalassemia
Spherocytes:	Hereditary spherocytosis Autoimmune hemolysis Hemoglobin C disorders (CC, SC) Severe burns
Ovalocytes:	Hereditary ovalocytosis Megaloblastic anemia Iron deficiency Thalassemia

ANEMIA: APPROACH TO WORKUP

Routine Data Base

The following is an appropriate routine data base in the initial evaluation of anemia.

        Hct
        Hgb
        MCV
        MCHC
        Reticulocyte count
        Fingerstick peripheral smear

(The MCH gives essentially the same information as the MCV.)

Approach

Attempt to classify the anemia on the basis of (1) cell size, (2) mechanism, and (3) patient problem list. Answer the following three questions.

1.   What is the MCV?

        The normal MCV varies depending on the method, but with automated methods is in the range of 82-98 fl (remember that an MCV calculated from manually determined Hcts and RBCs is much less reproducible and, therefore, less useful than an MCV determined by automated counters). It is helpful to use a broad normal range of 80-100 fl to classify the anemia as microcytic (MCV < 80 fl), normocytic (MCV = 80-100 fl) or <u>macrocytic</u> (MCV > 100 fl). This is a most helpful step in the approach to etiology, since anemias with abnormal MCVs are caused by only a few conditions (Chapters 2 and 3).

2. <u>What is the basic mechanism of the anemia</u>?

There are only three basic ways that anemia may develop:

- Decreased effective marrow <u>production</u>
- <u>Bleeding</u>
- <u>Hemolysis</u>

The following observations help to define mechanism:

a. <u>Reticulocyte Index</u>. The reticulocyte count is used to assess the appropriateness of the bone marrow response to anemia. It must be corrected for the anemia to give a value known as the reticulocyte index (see p. 29). Anemia with appropriate bone marrow response (reticulocytosis) suggests bleeding or hemolysis. Be aware that a recently treated production type anemia (e.g., iron deficiency) or the discontinuation of marrow suppression (e.g., withdrawal of alcohol) will also manifest appropriate reticulocytosis and mimic hemolysis or acute bleeding.

b. <u>The rate of Hct fall</u> may help in the assessment of mechanism. Total marrow shutdown of production in the absence of bleeding/ hemolysis will result in a Hct fall of no greater than 3-4 Hct points per week (1/120 of the red cell mass per day, since the normal red cell survival is around 120 days). A fall more rapid than this, in the absence of marked plasma volume changes, usually means bleeding or hemolysis.

Remember: anemia with an appropriate reticulocyte response in the absence of bleeding usually means hemolysis (much less common than bleeding).

3. <u>What anemias are associated with the problems noted on the problem list</u>?

For this purpose, race and sex should be considered as well. Women are frequently iron deficient; black patients may have hemoglobinopathies or glucose-6-phosphate dehydrogenase (G-6-PD) deficiency, etc. Table 1.5 lists recognized causes for anemia in various clinical disease states.

Table 1.5
Anemias Associated with Various Clinical States

Female: Iron deficiency

Blacks: G-6-PD deficiency, hemoglobinopathies, thalassemia

Mediterranean Origin: G-6-PD deficiency, thalassemia

Far East Origin: Hemoglobinopathies

Viral infections: Immune hemolysis. Decreased production

Bacterial Infection: Anemia of inflammation
                        Microangiopathic hemolysis
                        Oxidative hemolysis (G-6-PD deficiency)
                        Other hemolytic mechanisms

Malignancy: Microangiopathic hemolysis
               Immune hemolysis
               Decreased production

Alcoholic Liver Disease: Bleeding
                         Hypersplenism
                         Folate deficiency
                         Ethanol depression of production
                         Sideroblastic anemia
                         Iron deficiency
                         Hemolysis

Hyper- or Hypothyroidism: Decreased production
                             Pernicious anemia
                             Iron deficiency

Renal Failure: Decreased production
               Hemolysis
               Bleeding

Aortic Valve Replacement: Microangiopathic hemolysis

Malignant Hypertension: Microangiopathic hemolysis

Rheumatoid Syndromes: Anemia of inflammation
                         Iron deficiency
                         Immune hemolysis

Collagen Vascular Disease: Immune hemolysis
                              Anemia of inflammation
                                  (Continued on following page)

Table 1.5 Cont'd

Drugs:

    Aldomet: Immune hemolysis
    Quinine/quinidine: Immune hemolysis
    Penicillin: Immune hemolysis (rare)
    Butazolidin/Chloramphenicol: Dose-related marrow depression
                                    Idiosyncratic aplastic anemia
    Gold: Aplastic anemia
    Antituberculosis drugs: Sideroblastic anemia
    Dilantin: Megaloblastic anemia (folate)
            Pure red cell aplasia
    Sulfa: G-6-PD hemolysis

Summary

Classification on the basis of (1) MCV, (2) categorization of probable mechanism, and (3) consideration of possible cause raised by the problem list should then suggest further appropriate diagnostic evaluation.

REFERENCES

Gottfried EL: Erythrocyte indices with electronic counter. N Engl J Med 300:1277, 1979.
Pinkerton PH, Spence I, Ogalvie JC, et al: An assessment of the Coulter Counter model S. J Clin Pathol 23:68, 1970.
Williams WJ: Examination of the blood. In Hematology, ed 3, New York, McGraw Hill, 1983, p 9.

Chapter 2

Anemias with a Low MCV

For the most part an MCV < 80 fl limits the anemia to one of two diagnoses: <u>iron deficiency</u> or some type of <u>thalassemia</u>. The anemia of chronic inflammation may occasionally be associated with an MCV in the 70s but usually is normocytic. Some hemoglobinopathies are associated with a low MCV. Hemoglobin E is the most common of these. It is seen almost exclusively in people from Southeast Asia (Thailand, Cambodia, Malaysia, and Indonesia). Sideroblastic anemias are characterized by heterogenous red cells including a population of microcytic (and hypochromic) cells but the MCV is rarely decreased (frequently increased, see Chapter 5).

DIFFERENTIAL DIAGNOSIS

. Iron deficiency

. Thalassemia

. Anemia of chronic disease (Chapter 5)

. Some hemoglobinopathies (e.g., Hgb E)

. Sideroblastic anemia (congenital, MCV rarely low, Chapter 5)

IRON DEFICIENCY ANEMIA

Dietary iron deficiency anemia may develop in the infant and adolescent because growth needs outstrip dietary supply. In some countries diets are so inadequate that dietary iron deficiency anemia develops in adults as well. However, in the United States iron deficiency on the basis of diet alone in an adult is uncommon. In adults one should essentially always consider iron deficiency to be secondary to blood loss. Iron deficiency in a man means gastrointestinal (GI) bleeding until proven otherwise. Fifty percent of young women are iron deficient because of menstrual bleeding and pregnancy.

History

The following historical data suggest iron deficiency:

- Any menstruating woman, especially with past pregnancies.

- Pica: ice, starch (Argo), clay ingestion.

- Postgastrectomy for bleeding without adequate postoperative iron supplementation.

- Any past history of GI bleeding.

Physical Findings

Sore tongue, cheilosis, brittle and ridged fingernails, spoon nails, and splenomegaly are all features of severe and long-standing iron deficiency anemia but are seen infrequently. Iron deficiency is associated rarely with an esophageal web (Plummer-Vinson syndrome).

The MCV is Usually Low

When blood loss occurs slowly but consistently over months, progressive anemia develops once the reticuloendothelial iron stores (approximately 1 g of iron in an adult) have been utilized. Initially red cell size and shape are unaffected, but as the anemia progresses cells become smaller and later misshapen. In general the MCV and degree of poikilocytosis correlate with the degree of anemia (Table 2.1).

Table 2.1		
Correlation of Hct, MCV and Shape Changes in Iron Deficiency Anemia		
Hct (%)	MCV (fl)	Poikilocytosis
35	82	0
30	79	1+
25	74	2+
20	70	3+
15	65	4+

The MCV Can Be Normal

- Early, mild iron deficiency anemia.

- When blood loss occurs rapidly over days to weeks, the bone marrow can produce normocytic red cells while iron stores are adequate.

Therefore, the MCV will often be normal despite a low hematocrit during early blood loss.

• Combined deficiencies of iron plus folate or B12.

• Early iron deficiency in patients with macrocytosis of liver disease.

The MCHC Is Usually Normal

Hypochromia develops as the anemia increases. However, the MCHC which reflects chromicity ordinarily does not drop until the hematocrit is quite low. In the past, when hematocrits were primarily determined by manual centrifugation techniques, significant plasma trapping occurred in iron deficiency anemia due to the deformed RBCs. This resulted in an erroneously high Hct and an early drop in the MCHC as anemia developed (MCHC = Hgb ÷ Hct). With the use of electronic counters it is unusual to see an abnormal MCHC in iron deficiency until the Hgb is less than 9 or 10 g%.

Other Diagnostic Aids In Iron Deficiency

• Serum iron (SI). Classically low, but also low in acute and chronic inflammation and malignancy.

• Total iron-binding capacity (TIBC). A measure of transferrin in terms of amount of iron it can bind, the TIBC is classically elevated, but is actually normal in many patients with iron deficiency. It is low in chronic inflammation and malignancy.

• Reticulocyte index. Inappropriately low for the degree of anemia (see p. 29).

• Serum ferritin. Low in moderate or severe iron deficiency anemia. May be in the low normal range in iron deficiency without anemia or with very mild anemia (see p. 13).

• Bone marrow iron stain. Absent iron stores in iron deficiency. A small amount of bone marrow iron may occasionally be seen when iron deficiency anemia develops in the setting of chronic inflammatory states (e.g., rheumatoid arthritis). Reticuloendothelial cell iron is present but unavailable for bone marrow use (p. 48).

• Peripheral smear. In early iron deficiency the smear is usually normal. It is difficult to pick up early subtle changes in cell size in early iron deficiency (microcytosis precedes poikilocytosis) and the MCV is more helpful than the smear at this stage. In severe iron deficiency anemia there is marked poikilocytosis and hypochromia without stippling. Elliptical ("cigar-shaped") cells are common. The few young cells seen on the smear frequently appear as polychromatophilic target cells.

. <u>Miscellaneous</u>. Either thrombocytosis or mild thrombocytopenia as well as leukopenia may occasionally be seen in severe iron deficiency anemia.

Common Appropriate Data Base

Most iron deficiency anemias may be diagnosed on the basis of history, the MCV, peripheral smear and the serum ferritin concentration.

Table 2.2
Representative Date Bases at Various Stages in the Slow Development
of Severe Iron Deficiency Anemia

Hct	42	42	35	27	19
MCV (82–98 fl)	92	88	81	75	68
MCHC (32–36g/dl)	33	33	33	33	29
SI (65–175 µg%)	70	60	35	20	20
TIBC (250–375 µg%)	300	300	300	400	450
Serum ferritin (10–200 µg/ml)	60	30	5	3	1
Peripheral smear	Normal	Normal	Normal	1+ poikilo-cytosis 1+ hypochromia	4+ poikilo-cytosis 4+ hypochromia
Bone marrow iron stores	Present	Absent	Absent	Absent	Absent

The Serum Ferritin

The serum ferritin has become a useful clinical measure of reticulo-endothelial iron stores. In general the serum ferritin level gives the same clinical information as a bone marrow iron stain. However, there are a number of exceptions which must be considered in the clinical use of this test. Table 2.3 lists conditions associated with serum ferritin levels which frequently are higher than are appropriate for the amount of reticuloendothelial iron present. In these conditions patients with iron deficiency anemia may have normal or even elevated serum ferritin levels.

Table 2.3
Inappropriately Normal or Elevated Serum Ferritin Levels

Acute liver disease
Cirrhosis
Hodgkin's disease
Acute leukemias
Solid tumors (occasional)
Fever
Acute inflammation
Renal dialysis patients
Recent treatment with iron

In patients with the anemia of chronic inflammation the serum ferritin, for the most part, will distinguish those who are iron deficient as well. However, the normal range may have to be adjusted upward somewhat as inflammation may slightly elevate the serum ferritin level in iron deficient patients. The same situation applies to hemodialysis patients. A number of studies of dialysis patients have demonstrated that a serum ferritin less than 50-55 μg/L is highly suggestive of iron deficiency, whereas a level greater than 100 μg/L usually means iron stores are present. Acute inflammation or any febrile illness may raise the serum ferritin levels for several days. Patients receiving oral or parenteral (especially the latter) iron therapy may immediately normalize the serum ferritin levels, long before the iron stores are replaced.

Treatment Tips

Standard medical therapy consists of one oral iron tablet (there are 60 mg of elemental iron in one 300 mg FeSO4 tablet) t.i.d. on an empty stomach (1 hour before meals). Treatment may need to be continued for a long time (1 year in a menstruating woman, 6 months in a man) to replenish iron stores. Avoid time-release spansules and enteric coated preparations (absorption is variable). The addition of ascorbic acid (to aid absorption) is not worth the cost. Although iron absorption is decreased in patients with achlorhydria or patients who are postgastrectomy, treatment with oral iron is still usually successful.

Patient compliance is the major problem with oral iron therapy. Approximately 15% of patients have GI side effects from oral iron (cramping, constipation, diarrhea). The following compromises may help compliance:

1. B.i.d. treatment rather than t.i.d. The middle of the day dose is difficult for patients to take.

2. Once a day for a year is better than b.i.d. or t.i.d. for 6 weeks.

3. If GI side effects occur, try the following:

    a. Administer the iron with meals (decrease absorption 50%), but not with antacids and not with tea (markedly decreases absorption).

    b. If symptoms still continue, decrease the size of each dose to less than 40 mg elemental iron. (Pediatric liquid preparations are frequently well tolerated.) Try on an empty stomach; if not tolerated, administer with meals.

4. Parenteral iron is rarely necessary if the above compromises are tried. Parenteral iron is indicated in patients with small and large bowel inflammation, rapid transit GI problems, malabsorption and proven noncompliance, or when time to respond is an urgent issue (e.g., third trimester and severe anemia). Side effects from parenteral iron include:

    .   Pain at the injection site

    .   Staining of the skin

    .   Fever

    .   Exacerbation of arthritis

    .   Anaphylaxis (very rare)

Treatment Response

The maximal reticulocyte response is seen 7-10 days following initiation of oral iron therapy. Reticulocyte counts on either side of the peak reticulocyte response may not be very high, especially if the anemia is not severe. The hematocrit will begin to rise 7-10 days following initiation of treatment at a rate inversely proportional to the degree of anemia.

THALASSEMIA

The thalassemias are inherited defects in globin chain production resulting in microcytic anemia. They are seen in the United States primarily in black patients and patients of Mediterranean (Greek or Italian) or Asian extraction. Most patients are heterozygotes and have mild, usually clinically asymptomatic, anemias but marked red cell microcytosis. Diagnosis is important in order to distinguish from iron deficiency (patients are frequently worked up repetitively for iron deficiency and treated with iron) and for genetic counseling.

Typical Routine Data Base Results for Heterozygous Thalassemia

Hematocrit	37
MCV	69
MCH	21
MCHC	33
Reticulocytes	3%
Smear:	microcytosis; moderate anisocytosis and poikilocytosis; occasional target cells, ovalocytes and coarsely stippled red cells.

This data base should stimulate the following question:

WHY IS THE MCV SO LOW FOR SUCH A MILD ANEMIA?

This question should suggest a diagnosis of heterozygous thalassemia. Typically, the MCV is in the 60s or low 70s but the hematocrit is normal or only slightly decreased. In iron deficiency an MCV this low is usually seen only with severe anemia (see p. 10). The occasional heavily stippled red cell on peripheral smear is also helpful in differentiating the disorder from iron deficiency. Such cells are more common in Greek or Italian patients than in the black patient with thalassemia. The polycythemic patient (especially polycythemia vera) with iron deficiency may have a hematologic data base which may mimic thalassemia.

Differential Diagnosis

1. Thalassemia

2. Polycythemia with iron deficiency

Further Data Base

In the normal adult three major hemoglobins are present in mature red cells. Each hemoglobin molecule consists of four heme groups and four globin chains. The globin chain in each hemoglobin molecule are of two different types. From the following table one sees that all these hemoglobins share one type of common globin chain (α chains), but differ in the type of the second globin chain (β, δ, γ):

Hemoglobin	%	Globin chain type
A	97%	$\alpha\,2\,\beta\,2$
A$_2$	2%	$\alpha\,2\,\delta\,2$
F	1%	$\alpha\,2\,\gamma\,2$

Hemoglobin electrophoresis. In heterozygous β-thalassemia there is decreased production of β globin chains, resulting in a decreased production of hemoglobin A, and a compensatory increase in δ globin chain production, resulting in an increase of Hgb A_2 ($3\frac{1}{2}$- 6%).

Assay of Hgb F. In heterozygous β-thalassemia there may also be a compensatory increase in production of γ globin chains, resulting in an increase of Hgb F (2-8%, present in about 50% of patients).

Miscellaneous. Other test results may help to distinguish thalassemia from iron deficiency (normal or elevated serum ferritin, the presence of iron on a bone marrow iron stain, and normal or elevated serum iron).

WHAT IF THALASSEMIA IS SUSPECTED BUT HGB A_2 IS NOT INCREASED?

Possible Explanation

1. Concomitant β-thalassemia and iron deficiency (the reason for the reduction of A_2 Hgb is not clear).

2. β-δ-thalassemia. This syndrome commonly results in a slightly more severe anemia, a normal or low hemoglobin A_2 and an increased hemoglobin F.

3. α-thalassemia. β-thalassemia syndromes are the most common form of thalassemia in American white populations of Mediterranean background, and approximately 1% of American blacks have β-thalassemia. α-thalassemia is more common in American blacks (as high as 30% incidence of heterozygous α-thalassemia). α chains are present in all three normal adult hemoglobins. Therefore, decreased α globin chain production does not alter the ratio of the three hemoglobins. Proof of α-thalassemia requires special research laboratory techniques or in-depth family studies. The genetics of α chain production are more complicated than for β chain production, and this results in significant variability in the severity of the clinical syndromes depending on the number (and type) of inherited gene defects.

    .   1 gene: Clinically silent.

    .   2 genes: A clinical syndrome resembling heterozygous β-thalassemia but with a normal Hgb electrophoresis.

    .   3 genes: Hgb H disease. Moderately severe anemia with Hgb H (β_4) inclusion in the red cells.

    .   4 genes: Death in utero ("hydrops fetalis").

Clinical Management

- **Patient education.** Explain that the clinical features mimic iron deficiency. Put patients on guard to protect themselves from iron deficiency workups. Emphasize the benign nature of the illness in heterozygotes. Explain that the anemia, being mild, does not usually cause symptoms (an Hct of 35% does not explain fatigue).

- **Caution** against taking oral iron.

- **Genetic counseling.** A couple, both heterozygous for β-thalassemia, have a 25% chance of having a child with homozygous thalassemia (thalassemia major, "Cooley's anemia"). The gene defects for thalassemia and those for Hgb S and Hgb C are alleles. Hgb S-thalassemia is a clinically significant disease (see p. 60). It is now possible to make a prenatal diagnosis of some thalassemia syndromes by amniocentesis.

- **Thalassemia major.** These patients require specialized treatment and should be followed by physicians experienced in their care.

REFERENCES

Benz EJ, Forget BG: The thalassemia syndromes: models for the molecular analysis of human disease. Annu Rev Med 33:363-373, 1982.

Blank A: The thalassemia syndromes. Blood 51:369-384, 1978.

England JM, Fraser PM: Differentiation of iron deficiency from thalassemia trait by routine blood count. Lancet 1:449-452, 1973.

England JM, Ward SM, Down MC: Microcytosis, anisocytosis and the red cell indices in iron deficiency. Br J Haematol 34:589-597, 1976.

Fairbanks UF: Is the peripheral blood film reliable for the diagnosis of iron deficiency anemia? Am J Clin Pathol 55:447-451, 1971.

Holliday JW, Powell LW: Serum ferritin and isoferritins in clinical medicine. In Progress in Hematology. New York, Grune and Stratton, 1979, Vol II, p. 229.

Kazazian HH, et al: Prenatal diagnosis of β-thalassemia by amniocentesis. Blood 56:926-930, 1980.

Rawley PT: The diagnosis of beta-thalassemia trait: a review. Am J Hematol 1:129-137, 1976.

Ward PCJ: Investigation of microcytic anemia. Postgrad Med 65:235-242, 1979.

Chapter 3

Anemias with a High MCV

An MCV greater than 100 fl needs to be explained. The differential diagnosis of the common etiologies is short. Some causes, such as marked reticulocytosis and macrocytosis seen in the newborn, are obvious from the routine data base. Further diagnostic studies may be necessary to distinguish megaloblastic anemia from the syndrome of preleukemia or from severe liver disease, as well as to define the specific etiology of a megaloblastic anemia once that diagnosis is made. The following is a list of common causes of an MCV greater than 100. Note that a number of these causes are not associated with anemia.

DIFFERENTIAL DIAGNOSIS OF AN MCV GREATER THAN 100 FL

1. Spurious
2. Reticulocytosis (marked)
3. Liver disease
4. Alcoholism
5. No associated disease
6. Refractory anemia (preleukemia, sideroblastic anemia)
7. Drugs
8. Megaloblastic anemias

1. A number of technical factors may contribute to a spurious elevation of the MCV as measured by the electronic counters. These include low temperature and inadequate removal of the bleach solution used to clean the system. Marked hyperglycemia or chronic hypernatremia will result in cell swelling when cells are placed in the more hypotonic counting solution. High titer "cold" and "warm" red cell autoantibodies may, on occasion, by agglutination, cause spuriously high MCVs.

2. Young red cells are large and will elevate the average MCV. Reticulocyte counts must be quite high to increase the MCV over 100 fl. It is uncommon to see an MCV greater than 115 fl from reticulocytosis alone.

3. Hepatocellular and obstructive liver disease is frequently associated

18

with an elevated MCV (usually less than 110 fl). In liver disease the red cell membrane accumulates lipid. The cells appear large, round and targeted on smear, without the marked variation in size and shape characteristic of megaloblastic anemia. This morphologic abnormality is not an explanation for anemia, although patients with liver disease frequently have anemia from other mechanisms.

4. Even without evidence of liver disease or a megaloblastic anemia, the severe alcoholic frequently has a mildly elevated MCV (100-110 fl). The cause of the elevated MCV is unclear, but it has been well documented to occur in the absence of any evidence of liver disease or folate deficiency. There is a correlation between the degree of elevation of the MCV and the amount of alcohol consumption. It goes away slowly (2-4 months) on discontinuation of alcohol intake.

5. Occasionally one sees a mild elevation of the MCV (100-105 fl) in a patient without any known cause.

6. Refractory anemia with hyperplastic bone marrow (preleukemia, sideroblastic anemia, etc., p. 20, 50).

7. A number of drugs cause mild to severe megaloblastic bone marrow changes with associated peripheral macrocytosis. Drugs such as alcohol and diphenylhydantoin interfere with folate utilization and/or absorption. Methotrexate and trimethoprim bind to dihydro-folate reductase, interfering with folate metabolism. Other chemotherapeutic agents, such as cytosine arabinoside and hydroxyurea, interfere with DNA metabolism, resulting in a hematologic defect which mimics folic acid deficiency. Chronic use of cyclophosphamide, 6-mercaptopurine, azathioprine, 5-fluorouracil and other chemotherapeutic agents results in a mild elevation of the MCV.

8. Megaloblastic anemia (p. 21)

HINTS AS TO ETIOLOGY FROM THE INITIAL ROUTINE DATA BASE

Common Historical and Physical Findings:

- Sore tongue, smooth tongue (megaloblastic anemia)

- Peripheral neuropathy, dorsal column signs, "megaloblastic madness," rarely corticospinal track signs, hypothyroidism or hyperthyroidism, postgastrectomy, ileal disease or resection (B12 deficiency).

- Alcoholic, marked inanition, malabsorption, Dilantin (folic acid deficiency or inhibition).

- Stigmata of liver disease.

Routine Laboratory Help

- An MCV greater than <u>115 fl</u> is unusual except in megaloblastic anemia.

- Marked variations in size (<u>anisocytosis</u>) and shape (<u>poikilo-cytosis</u>) with <u>ovalocytes</u> on smear are classically seen in severe megaloblastic anemia but may also be seen in the refractory anemias with hypercellular bone marrow (preleukemia, sideroblastic anemia, etc.)

- <u>Leukopenia</u> and <u>thrombocytopenia</u> are common in megaloblastic anemia and preleukemia but might also be seen in liver disease for different reasons (hypersplenism, alcohol).

- The <u>reticulocyte count</u> is inappropriately low in megaloblastic anemias and preleukemia.

- <u>Neutrophil hypersegmentation</u> is common in megaloblastic anemias (although not invariable), but is not seen in pre-leukemia.

- <u>Bizarre platelet morphology</u> and marked <u>qualitative white cell changes</u> favor a diagnosis of preleukemia.

- The macrocytes in liver disease are round and frequently <u>targeted</u> (not oval as in megaloblastic anemia).

FURTHER DATA BASE

If the etiology of the elevated MCV is not obvious after the above considerations, further diagnostic workup is indicated. That workup is usually directed at evaluation for the presence of a megaloblastic anemia and usually consists of:

1. Serum B12 assay
2. Serum folic acid assay
3. Bone marrow aspiration with iron stain

The further data should allow one to distinguish a megaloblastic anemia from the syndrome of preleukemia, which may mimic a megaloblastic process.

Preleukemia (Refractory Anemias with a Hypercellular Bone Marrow)

This syndrome is an acquired bone marrow stem cell disorder seen primarily in older patients. Frequently there are qualitative and quantitative abnormalities of all cell lines, and the picture may mimic closely a megaloblastic anemia. The MCV does not reach the levels seen in severe megaloblastic anemias and rarely is greater than 110 fl. The MCV may be normal. Red cells typically show marked anisocytosis and poikilocytosis with macro-ovalocytes, stippling and nucleated red cells. There may be leukopenia and thrombocytopenia. Platelets may appear large and degranulated, and there are usually qualitative white cell changes peripherally, frequently with an increase in young monocytes. Hypersegmentation of the polys is not seen. The bone marrow typically is hypercellular and there are qualitative changes in all cell lines, the erythrocyte precursors frequently appearing megaloblastic. White cell precursors reveal a left shift and are abnormal with clusters of young mononuclear forms. The iron stain frequently reveals ringed sideroblasts. The serum B12 and serum folate levels are typically high, and there is no response to treatment with folic acid or B12. With time (months to sometimes several years) such patients usually slowly develop a picture of acute leukemia. Some patients, however, develop worsening cytopenias leading to severe refractory anemia with a transfusion requirement, bleeding, or infection and death without evidence of overt acute leukemia.

<u>Various terms used to describe this syndrome</u>:

- Preleukemia
- Refractory anemia with an excess of blasts
- Smoldering leukemia
- Subacute leukemia
- Myelomonocytic leukemia syndrome
- Erythroleukemia
- Di Guglielmo syndrome

Megaloblastic Anemia

Table 3.1 lists the various causes of B12 and folic acid deficiency.

Table 3.1
Causes of Vitamin B12 and Folic Acid Megaloblastosis

B12

Pernicious anemia (acquired and congenital)
Gastrectomy
Ileal resection
Crohn's disease and tropical sprue
Fish tapeworm infestation
Blind loop syndrome
Nutritional deficiency (vegan's diet, rare)
Familial selective malabsorption (Imerslund's syndrome)

(Continued on following page)

Table 3.1 Cont'd.

Folic Acid

Dietary (old age, the alcoholic, chronic disease)
Malabsorption (sprue)
Hemodialysis
Severe exfoliative skin disease (e.g. psoriasis)
Drugs

   Interference with absorption or metabolism (Dilantin, alcohol)
   Dihydrofolate reductase inhibitors (methotrexate, trimethoprim)

Increased requirements

   Pregnancy
   Infancy
   Hemolysis (e.g., Sickle Cell Anemia)

History and Physical

Remember that pernicious anemia (PA) is by far the most common etiology of B12 deficiency. The body's store of B12 will last for years, and, therefore, dietary B12 deficiency is extremely rare. Patients may complain of sore mouth, indigestion, constipation or diarrhea. Neurologic problems (peripheral neuropathy, dorsal column signs, changes in affect) are common. Remember that the anemia develops so slowly that patients may be quite well compensated to very low hematocrits. Other causes of B12 deficiency are listed above. After total gastrectomy or total ileectomy, all patients will after many years develop B12 deficiency and megaloblastic anemia. Such patients should receive prophylactic B12 treatment. After partial gastrectomy only a rare patient develops B12 deficiency.

Table 3.2
Neurologic Features of B12 Deficiency

Peripheral neuropathy	(common)
Dorsal column signs	(relatively common)
Corticospinal tract signs	(rare)
"Megaloblastic madness"	(common)

In contrast to B12 deficiency, the body's stores of folic acid will last only a few weeks, and, therefore, folic acid deficiency is usually dietary. Folic acid deficiency is seen most commonly in the alcoholic or the patient with extremely poor food intake of several weeks' duration from any cause. The condition is also seen in the pregnant patient without prenatal care, and rarely in the patient with chronic hemolysis. The symptoms are those of B12 deficiency

but without the neurologic manifestations. Remember that the alcoholic
may have a neuropathy from alcohol.

Laboratory

Peripheral blood and bone marrow

Peripheral blood and bone marrow morphology is the same
in B12 and folic acid deficiency with moderate to severe anemia.
The MCV is frequently greater than 115 fl. If the anemia is
severe, red cells demonstrate marked anisocytosis and poikilocytosis,
with macro-ovalocytosis. There are, however, also small misshapen
cells. Howell-Jolley bodies (p. 5), Pappenheimer bodies (p. 5)
and nucleated RBCs may be seen. The neutrophils are frequently
hypersegmented (six or more lobes) and decreased in number.
(Note: A left shift in granulocytes, as with infection, or severe
neutropenia may mask hypersegmentation.) The hypersegmentation
usually persists for 10 days to 2 weeks after treatment. Platelets
may be decreased. The bone marrow is typically hypercellular
with megaloblastic abnormalities of erythroid and granulocytic
precursors. Iron stain of the marrow frequently reveals abnormal
sideroblasts, and even occasional ringed sideroblasts may be
seen.

Serum folate and B12 levels

In B12 deficiency (PA) the serum B12 level is usually quite
low and the serum folate level is usually normal or elevated
(low in 10% of patients). However, since the advent of radioimmune
dilution assays the serum B12 has become much less reliable than
with the old microbiologic assay resulting in falsely normal
results in some patients with PA. This problem is improving
with the more recent assay methods which utilize intrinsic factors,
rather than R-binders, as the binding protein. Following parenteral
B12 administration the serum B12 level may be elevated for weeks
eliminating it as a diagnostic tool for B12 deficiency.

In megaloblastic anemia due to folic acid deficiency the
serum folate is typically quite low. However, the serum folate
is so sensitive to recent dietary intake that it is of little
help in the diagnostic workup of megaloblastic anemia. The red
cell folate is a much better indicator of chronic folate deficiency.
The serum B12, although usually normal, may be low in up to 30%
of patients with folate deficient megaloblastic anemia. The
low B12 level is not due to a deficiency of B12 and normalizes
within a few days after beginning treatment with folic acid.

Table 3.3
Serum B12 Assay

1. Spuriously low in some patients with folate deficiency.
2. Spuriously low in some pregnant patients.
3. May be elevated for weeks after one shot of B12.
4. Increased in myeloproliferative syndromes.

RBC Folate Assay

1. Reflects chronic folate deficiency.
2. Falsely low in some patients with B12 deficiency.
3. Falsely high in reticulocytes.

Serum Folate Assay

1. A measure of recent dietary intake of folate.
2. Usually normal or elevated in B12 deficiency.

Table 3.4
Differentiating Between Folate and B12 Megaloblastosis

Etiology by History	RBC Folate	Serum B12	Interpretation	Further Testing
Suggests folate	↓	Nl or ↑	Folate Deficiency	None
Suggests folate	↓	Sl ↓	Folate Deficiency	Recheck B12 after folate Rx for 1 week
Suggests B12	Nl or ↑	↓	B12 Deficiency	None
Suggests B12	↓ (serum folate usually ↑)	↓	B12 Deficiency	May confirm with Schilling test

All other combinations → Schilling test.

Table 3.5
Causes of a Falsely Positive Schilling Test

1. Incomplete urine collection.
2. Renal failure
3. Some patients with megaloblastic anemia before treatment.
4. Gastric antibodies to intrinsic factor.
5. Defective intrinsic factor
6. Drugs (alcohol, colchicine, neomycin, potassium, cholestiramine)
7. Pancreatic insufficiency.

Schilling test

The Schilling test is of use primarily in cases in which there is confusion about the etiology of a megaloblastic anemia. Remember that the test requires a cooperative patient who can and will collect 24-hour urine samples. Also remember that the Schilling test may be abnormal initially in megaloblastic anemias (including folate deficiency) because of intestinal mucosal cell dysfunction secondary to the megaloblastic process. The Schilling test is more reliable after the megaloblastic anemia has been treated for 1-2 weeks.

Other laboratory features

Remember that megaloblastic anemias are hemolytic in the sense that there is marked intramarrow destruction of abnormally formed red cells (ineffective erythropoiesis). There is frequently indirect hyperbilirubinemia, elevated serum lactate dehydrogenase (LDH) and an elevated serum iron as in other hemolytic states. There is gastric achlorhydria in pernicious anemia. The reticulocyte index is inappropriately low. In PA antibodies to gastric mucosal cells and intrinsic factor are commonly found in the serum as well as antithyroid and antiadrenal antibodies.

Treatment

B12 deficiency

One hundred micrograms of intramuscular B12 monthly is adequate therapy for most patients. Many physicians will treat patients daily while they are in the hospital, especially if neurologic manifestations are prominent. However, there are few data to indicate that this is helpful. Patients with PA or after total gastrectomy or ileectomy should remain on monthly injections for life.

Folic acid deficiency

One milligram p.o. daily is adequate treatment for most

Table 3.6

Laboratory Features in Three Conditions Associated with an Elevated MCV

	Liver Disease	Megaloblastic anemia	Preleukemia
MCV	Usually <110 fl	Maybe >110 fl	Usually < 110 fl
WBCs	Variable	Frequently decreased	Frequently decreased
Platelets	Variable	Frequently decreased	Frequently decreased
RBC morphology	Targets No A and P	Marked A and P Macro-ovalocytes Tear drop cells	Marked A and P May mimic megalo-blastic anemia
NRBs	Not common	Common	Common
WBC morphology	Normal	Hypersegmented	Abnormal mononuclear cells, no hyper-segmentation
Platelet morphology	Normal	Normal	Frequently large and degranulated
Serum folate	Depends on diet	Decreased in folate deficiency; elevated in B12 deficiency	Normal or elevated
Serum B12	Normal	Decreased in B12 de-ficiency; may be slightly decreased in folate deficiency	Normal or elevated

patients. Alcoholics may require more (5 mg daily). Patients with chronic severe hemolytic states (e.g., sickle cell anemia) should receive prophylactic folic acid (1 mg per day).

Therapeutic trial

B12 or folic acid in the above doses will correct (at least partially) the megaloblastic anemia due to deficiency of the other vitamin. Occasionally in confusing cases therapeutic trials may be helpful diagnostically. One microgram of B12 i.m. will cause a reticulocytosis in B12 deficiency, but not in folate deficiency. Fifty micrograms of folic acid p.o. or parenterally will cause a reticulocytosis in folic acid deficiency, but not in B12 deficiency.

Response to therapy

With appropriate treatment of B12 and folic acid deficiency there is a rapid reticulocytosis which reaches its peak at about 7 days. The height of the reticulocyte response depends on the severity of the anemia. When the hematocrit is very low, the reticulocyte response may be 30 or 40% in the absence of other processes which blunt bone marrow response (inflammatory illness, etc.). The leukopenia and thrombocytopenia usually respond rapidly (in a few days). In PA, "megaloblastic madness" usually corrects rapidly; dorsal column disease and peripheral neuropathies usually improve, but more slowly. Corticospinal tract signs are usually permanent.

Transfusions

Some patients with a megaloblastic process may develop a very severe anemia. This is especially common in pernicious anemia. Resist the temptation to transfuse the elderly patient with PA just because the hematocrit is 10 or 15%. Such patients have developed the anemia very slowly and frequently are well compensated (including an expanded total blood volume). Transfusion, even of packed cells, may precipitate pulmonary edema. If comfortable at bed rest, it is best, if possible, to treat with the appropriate vitamin (or both if the etiology is not clear) and avoid the hazard of transfusion. If transfusion is necessary (see below), consider exchange transfusion to prevent increasing the blood volume or concomitant treatment with diuretics.

Major Indications for Transfusion

1. Angina
2. Ischemic changes on electrocardiogram
3. High output heart failure

Serum potassium

Frequently the serum potassium falls with treatment of a severe megaloblastic anemia, and cardiac arrhythmias related to hypokalemia with death have rarely been reported. Monitor the serum potassium closely and supplement if needed.

REFERENCES

Bennet JM, Catovsky D, Daniel MT: Proposals for the classification of the myelodysplastic syndromes. Br J Haematol 51:189, 1981.

Davidson RJL, Hamilton PJ: High mean red cell volume: its incidence and significance in routine hematology. J Clin Pathol 31:493, 1978.

Eichner ER: The hematologic disorders of alcoholism. Am J Med 54:621, 1973.

Hoffbrand AV, ed. Clinics in Haematology: Megaloblastic Anaemia. Philadelphia, WB Saunders, 1978.

Lawson DH, Parker JLW, Murray RM, et al: Hypokalemia in megaloblastic anaemias. Lancet 558, 1970.

Lindenbaum J: Folate and vitamin B12 deficiencies in alcoholism. Sem in Hematol 17:119-129, 1980.

Lindenbaum J, Pezzimenti JF, Shea N: Small intestinal function in vitamin B12 deficiency. Ann Intern Med 80:326, 1974.

McPhedran P, Bannes MG, Weinstein JS, et al: Interpretation of electronically determined macrocytosis. Ann Intern Med 78:677, 1973.

Chapter 4

Hemolysis and Bleeding: Anemia with a Normal or Slightly Elevated MCV and an Appropriate Reticulocyte Index

Anemia due to hemolysis or bleeding is characterized by the presence of a reticulocytosis indicating an appropriate bone marrow response. The MCV is usually normal, although mild elevation is not uncommon when the reticulocyte count is markedly elevated (see p. 18). A reticulocyte count should be part of the routine data base. It is used to assess the appropriateness of the bone marrow response to the anemia. An anemia with an appropriate reticulocyte response in the absence of overt bleeding suggests hemolysis.

Remember:

1. The normal reticulocyte count in a patient with a normal Hct is 1%. Approximately 1% of circulating RBCs are removed daily and replaced by marrow reticulocytes (approximately 20 cc of RBCs per day in an adult).

2. The marrow can triple its production of RBCs almost immediately in response to acute blood loss or hemolysis.

3. If hemolysis is chronic (months to years), the marrow production may reach a level of production greater than 10 times normal.

RETICULOCYTE INDEX

In order for the reticulocyte count to be used as an indicator of marrow responsiveness, it must be corrected for the anemia. This corrected reticulocyte count is known as the reticulocyte index.

$$\text{reticulocyte index} = \text{reticulocyte \% X } \frac{\text{patient Hct}}{\text{normal Hct}}$$

In anemia, with the same amount of bone marrow production, the percentage of reticulocytes increases because the reticulocytes are diluted in fewer red cells. This gives a false impression of increased bone marrow responsiveness. When the bone marrow response to anemia is appropriate, the reticulocyte index should be at least 3%.

Example

Hct 10%   reticulocyte count 5%

reticulocyte index = 5% X $\frac{10}{50}$ = 1%

In this example (which uses for ease of calculation an arbitrary normal Hct of 50%) there is an inappropriately low reticulocyte index, indicating that bone marrow production is at least a contributing factor in the etiology of anemia. The elevated reticulocyte count of 5% is misleading. For this degree of anemia an appropriate reticulocyte count would be at least 15%:

reticulocyte index = 15% X $\frac{10}{50}$ = 3%

THE "SHIFT" PHENOMENON

Young very large reticulocytes, which ordinarily remain in the bone marrow 2 or 3 days before release, are shifted out of the marrow early into the peripheral blood under the stimulus of high levels of erythropoietin. Such "shift cells" are especially common when the anemia is severe and develops rapidly. This phenomenon explains the very high reticulocyte counts frequently seen in acute and marked anemias. Remember that high reticulocyte counts, especially when many "shift cells" are present, may result in an elevated MCV.

THINK OF HEMOLYSIS WHEN:

1. Anemia is accompanied by an appropriate reticulocyte index in the absence of evidence of bleeding. But remember the following pitfalls:

    a. Patients with production anemias (as in iron deficiency, folate deficiency, marked alcoholism, infection) will sometimes experience a marked reticulocytosis in response to treatment (iron, folate, ethanol withdrawal, antibiotics), resulting in a laboratory data base which may mimic hemolysis.

    b. There may be marked silent internal blood loss (e.g., retroperitoneal bleeding in a patient on anticoagulation, or bleeding at the site of a hip fracture) which may mimic hemolysis. Bleeding is infinitely more common than hemolysis. Always suspect occult bleeding. Recognize the marked amount of blood loss through phlebotomy that may occur during a prolonged hospitalization.

2. Hemolysis is also suggested by a hematocrit which falls

rapidly over a few days, in the absence of bleeding. If red cell survival is normal, complete shutdown of marrow production results in a hematocrit drop at a normal rate of only 4-5% per week. A fall at a faster rate suggests bleeding or hemolysis.

APPROACH TO HEMOLYSIS

Before any attempt to define the specific etiology, it is reasonable first to attempt to prove hemolysis as the mechanism for the anemia. Further appropriate diagnostic tests will vary depending on whether one suspects an intravascular or extravascular mechanism.

Intravascular Hemolysis

When RBC destruction is rapid and occurs primarily within the vascular space, diagnosis is relatively easy. One sees the following:

1. Hemoglobinemia: Although one may measure the plasma hemoglobin level directly, visual inspection alone is useful. Plasma serum becomes visibly red or brown at a low level of Hgb (around 30 mg%), a level which occurs from the lysis of only a few milliliters of red cells. Remember that the simple screening tests for hemoglobin (e.g., Hemoccult) are too sensitive to be helpful in this determination, as there is normally a low level of free plasma hemoglobin from the trauma of drawing and centrifuging blood.

2. Hemoglobinuria occurs once haptoglobin (see below) is saturated (Hgb-haptoglobin complex is too large to pass the glomerulus and is cleared by the reticuloendothelial system) and may be suspected by visual inspection of the urine (red or brown). Occult blood in the urine in the absence of any microscopic hematuria is suggestive of hemoglobinuria but does not distinguish it from myoglobinuria. Because myoglobin is a small molecule it freely passes through the glomerulus, resulting in red or brown urine without plasma coloration. The larger hemoglobin molecule accumulates in the plasma before passing into the urine, resulting in red or brown coloration of both.

3. Saturation of haptoglobin (a binding protein for hemoglobin produced in the liver) occurs rapidly with an appreciable hemoglobinemia. Measurement of free haptoglobin is, therefore, a useful test in hemolysis. However, results frequently are not available for several days.

4. Hemosiderinuria (iron seen within renal tubular cells on an iron stain of the urinary sediment) is seen several days after the hemolytic event. Free hemoglobin (containing iron) passes the glomerulus and is absorbed by renal tubular

cells, which slough, appear in the urine several days later and stain positively for iron.

Table 4.1
Clinical States Associated with Intravascular Hemolysis

1. Acute hemolytic transfusion reactions.
2. Severe and extensive burns.
3. Physical trauma (e.g., March hemoglobinuria).
4. Severe microangiopathic hemolysis (e.g., aortic valve prosthesis).
5. Acute G-6-PD hemolysis.
6. Paroxysmal nocturnal hemoglobinuria.
7. Clostridial sepsis.

Thus an appropriate further data base when hemolysis is suspected in the above clinical settings would include:

1. Observation of the serum/plasma.

2. Observation of the urine.

3. Measurement of free plasma hemoglobin.

4. Heme pigment test of the urine if there are no red cells in the urine sediment.

5. Measurement of free serum haptoglobin.

6. Iron stain of urine sediment for hemosiderin several days after a presumed hemolytic event.

Do not forget the help that may be obtained from the peripheral smear (p. 33).

Extravascular Hemolysis

Most hemolytic events do not take place intravascularly. When destruction occurs primarily within phagocytic cells of the reticuloendothelial system (RES), diagnosis is more difficult. There is no hemoglobinemia, hemoglobinuria or hemosiderinuria. Haptoglobin is only partially saturated (there is usually a slight leak of free hemoglobin into the circulation even when hemolysis is primarily occurring extravascularly). There may be an indirect hyperbilirubinemia (insensitive) and an increase in the urine urobilinogen (unreliable). Red cells are rich in lactic dehydrogenase, which is frequently elevated in the serum. However, the test is too nonspecific and too often spurious (from the trauma of drawing and processing blood) to be useful. The RBC survival is shortened, but this test is tedious and takes days to complete. In short, the physician must frequently be satisfied

with only presumptive evidence of extravascular hemolysis. When extravascular hemolysis is suspected, it is appropriate to move on to <u>diagnostic
tests of specific hemolytic states</u> based on possible etiologies from
the problem list and baseline data base without an absolute proof
of hemolysis. Most clinical hemolytic states are associated with
<u>extravascular</u> hemolysis.

Table 4.2
Common Clinical States Associated with Extravascular Hemolysis

1. Autoimmune hemolysis,
2. Delayed hemolytic transfusion reactions.
3. Hemoglobinopathies.
4. Hereditary spherocytosis.
5. Hypersplenism.
6. Hemolysis with liver disease.

Help from the Peripheral Smear

. Frequently the smear only reveals <u>evidence of bone marrow response</u>
(polychromatophilia, "shift cells," fine diffuse stippling).

. Occasionally individual red cell morphology suggests an etiology,
but frequently the morphology is <u>normal</u>. <u>There is no such thing
as a "hemolytic smear."</u> When present the following cell types
are helpful.

1. <u>Spherocytes</u>

    In small numbers, these are seen in many different etiologies.
    In large numbers, they suggest:

    a. Hereditary spherocytosis.
    b. Autoimmune hemolysis.
    c. Hgb C hemoglobinopathies (CC, SC, C-thalassemia).

2. <u>Elliptocytes/ovalocytes</u>

    Hereditary elliptocytosis.

3. <u>Fragmentation</u> (schistocytes)

    Sharply pointed poikilocytes (helmet cells, spiculated cells,
    triangle cells) seen in microangiopathic hemolytic states
    (see p. 40).

4. <u>Spiculated cells</u>

    Sometimes seen in patients with severe liver disease and
    hemolysis (usually seen only in patients with end-stage,

terminal liver disease). Also one of the types of schistocytes seen in microangiopathic hemolysis.

5. **"Bite" cells ("blister" cells)**

    Cells sometimes seen in patients with oxidative hemolysis (e.g., G-6-PD deficiency with hemolysis). In such cells all of the hemoglobin appears to be pushed to one side of the cell.

6. Poikilocytosis of the hemoglobinopathies (see p. 46).

HEMOLYSIS WITH A POSITIVE COOMBS' TEST

Once the physician suspects hemolysis from the above considerations, further diagnostic exploration should be guided by the routine data base and the problem list. Because of the reasonably common occurrence of immune hemolysis and the important therapeutic implications of this diagnosis, a Coombs' test is frequently obtained at this point if the etiology is not apparent.

Positive Coombs' Test: Serologic Questions

The serologic questions raised by finding a positive direct Coombs' test are the following:

1. **What exactly is on the surface of the red cell causing the positive test?**

    A screening direct Coombs' test usually employs nonspecific Coombs' antiserum (harvested from animals immunized with whole human serum) which will cause red cell agglutination if any one of a number of serum constituents are present on the cell. Specific Coombs' antisera allow the blood bank technician to distinguish among the following possibilities:

    a. **Transferrin:** Present on the surface of reticulocytes; therefore, marked reticulocytosis may cause a **weakly positive** direct Coombs' test with the use of broad-spectrum Coombs' antiserum. The direct Coombs' test using specific anti-IgG or anti-C3 will be negative.

    b. **Nonspecific protein binding:** Sometimes seen, for example in patients receiving high doses of the cephalosporins (negative Coombs' with specific antisera).

    c. **Complement:** Present in many cases of antibody-induced hemolysis. Complement may be present alone without an identifiable antibody. Its presence implies the presence of antibody no longer on the red cell or present in too low a concentration to identify.

d. Antibody: For the most part these are IgG antibodies, as
    Coombs' antisera do not contain anti-IgM or anti-IgA in
    significant concentration.

2. If antibody is present or presumed (complement alone), is it
    an alloantibody or an autoantibody?

Alloantibodies

- Induced by exposure to foreign red cells (transfusion
  or through pregnancy).

- Directed against specific minor red cell antigens.

- Present in the serum and identified by an antibody
  screen ("indirect Coombs' Test").

- Present on red cells (positive direct Coombs' test)
  only when transfused or fetal red cells are circulating,
  having been sensitized but not yet destroyed.

The blood bank can identify the specificity of such antibodies
by the pattern of reactivity seen using the patient's serum
and a panel of red cells of known and variable individual
antigenicity. Alloantibodies react only with some of the
cells (those containing the guilty antigen), as opposed
to the pan-reactivity of autoantibodies. Occasionally the
blood bank reports a positive antibody screen due to a naturally
occurring antibody. Such antibodies are not induced by
prior exposure to foreign red cells but may be quite hemolytic
if incompatible blood is transfused.

Clinical Significance

It is crucial to identify the presence and specificity
of such antibodies in order to assure the safety of future
transfusions. The difficulty of finding compatible blood
relates to the prevalence of the specific offending antigen
or antigens. The physician must communicate closely with
the blood bank to understand the problems the technician
faces in finding compatible blood.

Recommendation:

Pocket slide indicators containing information about
specific alloantibodies, the chance of finding compatible
blood, and how likely the antibody is to cause a transfusion
reaction are available through most blood banks and are
helpful to the house officer attempting to understand such
transfusion problems.

Autoantibodies:

A positive direct Coombs' test due to an antibody in a nonpregnant and not recently transfused patient is almost always due to an inappropriately produced autoantibody (immunologic defect, cross-reacting antibody secondary to drugs or infection, etc.). The antibody when eluted off the red cells (or if present also in the serum) reacts as a panagglutinin, reacting with all the cells in a routine red cell panel, making cross matching almost impossible.

Table 4.3
Alloantibody versus Autoantibody

	Alloantibody	Autoantibody
Direct Coombs'	Frequently negative. May be positive if sensitized foreign red cells are still circulating	Positive
Indirect Coombs'	Positive	Positive or negative
Antibody Screen (Panel)	Specificity is seen	Panagglutination no specificity seen

3. Once it is determined that the positive direct Coombs' is due to an autoantibody, the next serologic question is whether the antibody is a "warm antibody" or a "cold antibody."

    a. Warm Antibody

        . Usually IgG. Cannot be identified by direct agglutination (requires Coombs' test for identification).

        . Some IgG antibodies fix complement. Specific Coombs' antisera testing may reveal IgG alone, IgG plus C3 or, rarely, C3 alone.

    b. Cold Antibodies ("cold agglutinins")

        . Usually IgM and can be identified by direct agglutination in the cold. (Do not require Coombs' test for identification).

        . Positive "bedside cold agglutination test." Clumping may be seen by tilting a tube of the patient's anticoagulated blood in front of a light after placing it in a cup of ice water for 5 minutes.

- **Positive Coombs' test** due to C3 alone (positive "nongamma" Coombs'). IgM fixes C3 on the cell in the cold or at room temperature. IgM falls off on warming, but the C3 remains attached to the cell.

- Elevated <u>cold agglutinin titer</u>. Remember that we all normally have a low titer of naturally occurring cold agglutinins. An elevated titer is usually greater than 1:32 (read microscopically). Sera should be separated from the red cells immediately after drawing the blood while it is still warm in order not to lose antibody from adherence to the red cells as the blood cools to room temperature.

- The antibody usually is directed against a ubiquitous red cell antigen known as "I." Occasionally cold agglutinins (for example, those seen commonly in infectious mononucleosis) have a specificity for red cell antigen "i," which is present on newborn red cells.

Positive Coombs' Test: Clinical Questions

The clinical diagnostic and therapeutic considerations depend on the answers to the serologic questions discussed above. The clinical issues related to alloantibodies are discussed on p. 35.

AUTOIMMUNE HEMOLYSIS DUE TO A "WARM ANTIBODY"

Differential Diagnosis

A.   Idiopathic
B.   Secondary

Infection (particularly viral)
Drugs

Aldomet
Penicillin
Quinine/quinidine type

Collagen vascular disease (SLE)
Lymphoproliferative disorders
Miscellaneous (thyroid disease, malignancy, etc.)

Idiopathic Autoimmune Hemolysis

Many patients subsequently develop disease known to be associated with autoimmune hemolysis, such as SLE or lymphoma. Patients usually present with symptoms of anemia. the physical examination may reveal a slightly enlarged spleen (50% of cases). Jaundice and fever are

not common. The peripheral smear typically reveals marked polychromatophilia with "shift cells" and spherocytes. Usually the reticulocyte
count is markedly elevated; however, reticulocytopenia may be present
in some patients until after treatment, greatly confusing the diagnosis.
The white count and platelet count are usually normal or slightly
decreased, although rarely severe autoimmune thrombocytopenia may
be present as well (Evans' syndrome).

Secondary Autoimmune Hemolysis

Acute self-limited cases may be associated with various viral
illnesses or secondary to a number of drugs. A number of different
mechanisms have been described in hemolysis secondary to drugs.

1. ### Aldomet

    Seen in patients on large doses of Aldomet for several
    months. Usually there is only a positive Coombs' test without
    hemolysis. There is IgG alone on the surface of the red
    cell, and the serologic characteristics are exactly those
    seen in idiopathic (warm antibody) autoimmune hemolysis.
    The hematocrit returns to normal after the drug is stopped,
    although the direct Coombs' test may remain positive for
    months. In the absence of hemolysis, aldomet may be continued
    in patients with a positive Coombs' test alone.

2. ### Quinine/quinidine type

    Rare, but when seen usually presents with a fulminant
    hemolysis which may come soon after initiation of treatment.
    Antibody induced by the drug combines with the drug, and
    the immune complex deposits on the red cell. This is the
    common mechanism for hemolysis with a large number of other
    drugs which even more rarely may produce hemolysis.

3. ### Penicillin

    Again quite rare and more often seen in patients on
    massive doses of penicillin. The drug adheres to the surface
    of the red cell, occasionally inducing the formation of
    a hemolytic antibody. Note that this is not the common
    clinically unimportant antipenicillin antibody present in
    essentially all patients receiving the drug, and not the
    occasional antibody responsible for penicillin reactions.

Chronic cases of secondary Coombs'-positive hemolysis are seen
in patients with SLE (where the hemolysis may precede diagnosis by
months or years) and lymphoproliferative disorders (CLL, lymphosarcoma,
macroglobulinemia or Waldenstrom). Rarely Coombs'-positive hemolysis
may be associated with other malignancies, hyperthyroidism and various
bacterial infections.

AUTOHEMOLYSIS DUE TO COLD AGGLUTININ

Differential Diagnosis

1. Primary Cold Agglutinin Disease
2. Secondary

   a. Mycoplasma infections
   b. Viral infections
   c. Lymphoproliferative disease

The primary idiopathic form of the condition is quite rare, seen in elderly men, frequently with a monoclonal IgM serum protein electrophoretic spike, and symptoms, on occasion, of ischemia of the ears, nose and fingers in addition to anemia. Titers may be massively elevated.

Most commonly, cold agglutinin hemolysis is seen secondary to Mycoplasma or viral infections, SLE or lymphoproliferative disease. Fifty percent of patients with Mycoplasma pneumonia will have an elevated cold agglutinin titer (positive bedside test), but only a fraction of these have clinically significant hemolysis. Cold agglutinins (low titer with a specificity for the "i" antigen) are common in infectious mononucleosis, but significant hemolysis is rare.

TREATMENT

Acute Autoimmune Hemolysis

Acute Coombs'-positive hemolysis related to Mycoplasma or viral infections or to drugs requires only the discontinuation of the drug or time to recover from the infection.

Chronic Idiopathic Autoimmune Hemolysis (Warm Antibody)

Chronic Coombs'-positive hemolysis due to a warm antibody frequently responds to steroids. Prednisone in doses of 40-60 mg per day in divided doses is commonly employed. Response may take 1-3 weeks. The prednisone is then tapered slowly over several weeks. Most patients may be tapered off the steroid or to a small daily dose (2.5-10 mg prednisone per day). When hemolysis is severe and unresponsive to steroids or when the daily steroid dose is too high for safe long-term use, splenectomy should be considered. Immunosuppressive agents are usually reserved for the patient refractory to steroids and splenectomy. In many patients the disease is characterized by remissions and exacerbations over several years.

Secondary Autoimmune Hemolysis (Warm Antibody)

Secondary autoimmune hemolysis due to a warm antibody (SLE, CLL, lymphoma) may be more refractory to treatment (steroids and splenectomy) and responds best to successful control of the underlying disease process.

Cold Agglutinin Hemolysis

Steroids and splenectomy are much less successful in cold agglutinin hemolysis, although they are usually attempted. Protection from the cold may be helpful in chronic idiopathic cold agglutinin disease.

Transfusion Therapy

Transfusions may be necessary in these patients and present a problem, as compatible blood may be impossible to find. One should avoid transfusion if possible, but, if necessary, transfusion with ABO and Rh compatible blood may be attempted with close observation of the patient. Although the survival of the transfused cells is not normal, severe immediate intravascular hemolytic transfusion reactions are uncommon and there may be temporary improvement in the hematocrit. Small daily transfusions may be safer and more successful than large single transfusions. In patients with cold agglutinins it is reasonable to use blood that has been warmed to body temperature.

The major danger relates to the difficulty identifying a dangerous alloantibody in the setting of a warm autoantibody. The blood bank should attempt to hunt for hidden alloantibodies using special techniques (e.g., warm autoabsorption or a differential absorption technique). In addition, some warm autoantibodies have Rh specificity which is important to identify because transfused cells lacking the specific Rh antigen will survive longer.

HEMOLYSIS WITH FRAGMENTED RED CELLS ON PERIPHERAL SMEAR

Differential Diagnosis

Aortic valve replacement
Arteritis (malignant hypertension, polyarteritis, etc.)
Disseminated intravascular coagulation (DIC)
Thrombotic thrombocytopenic purpura (TTP)
Hemolytic uremic syndrome
Malignancy
Giant hemangiomas
Renal transplant rejection
Eclampsia

Data Base:

- The peripheral smear poikilocytosis is usually quite characteristic and may be differentiated from other conditions with marked poikilocytosis. The abnormal cells are sharply pointed and are called schistocytes. Common cell shapes include:

    helmet cell
    triangle cell

spiculated cell

- If hemolysis is severe it is usually intravascular, resulting in:

    Hemoglobinemia
    Hemoglobinuria
    Haptoglobin saturation
    Hemosiderinuria
    Iron deficiency if chronic (as with aortic valve
       prosthesis).

- If accompanied by significant thrombocytopenia think of DIC, hemolytic uremic syndrome, TTP or severe eclampsia. Thrombocytopenia is destructive, so there should be ample bone marrow megakaryocytes and large platelet forms on a fingerstick smear (p. 71).

HEMOLYSIS WITH AN ENLARGED SPLEEN

Although congestive splenomegaly is the most common cause, one may see cytopenias in patients with large spleens from any cause. All large spleens do not cause cytopenias, and the degree of cytopenia does not correlate with spleen size. Usually thrombocytopenia and leukopenia are more prominent than anemia. Red cell morphology is usually normal except for polychromatophilia and occasional spherocytes. Remember that splenomegaly is sometimes seen in patients with hemolysis from other mechanisms (e.g., autoimmune hemolysis, hereditary spherocytosis, etc.). One almost never has to consider splenectomy for hypersplenic cytopenias. Some patients with Felty's syndrome (complicated by recurrent infections from leukopenia) are benefited by splenectomy, as are occasional patients with chronic leukemia or lymphosarcoma.

HEMOLYSIS WITH LIVER DISEASE

Severe acute and chronic hepatocellular damage may be accompanied by hemolysis of unknown etiology. Occasionally one sees spiculated red cells (spur cells) on peripheral smear, a feature usually associated with severe hepatocellular disease and a very poor prognosis. Remember that patients with liver disease frequently have other mechanisms for anemia and reticulocytosis:

- Ethanol withdrawal may allow reticulocytosis in the alcoholic.

- A reasonable diet or folate replacement may result in a brisk reticulocytosis in the patient with alcoholic hepatitis and folate deficiency.

- Bleeding.

• Hypersplenism.

HEMOLYSIS WITH MICROSPHEROCYTES ON SMEAR

Differential Diagnosis

Hereditary spherocytosis (HS)
Coombs'-positive hemolysis (p. 34)
Hemoglobin C disorders (p. 60)
Severe burns

Data Base

• Spherocytes may be difficult to identify on peripheral smears
and require some experience to differentiate from a common
peripheral smear artifact. However, their presence in large
numbers suggests one of the above diagnoses.

Hereditary Spherocytosis

This is an autosomal dominant illness associated with microspherocytes
and polychromatophilia (large "shift cells" on smear) and a palpable
spleen. Mild jaundice is common. Severity is quite variable, and
some cases are not recognized until later in life. The condition
is due to an inherited red cell membrane defect. In vitro autohemolysis
in the absence of added glucose is accentuated, as is the osmotic
fragility of the cells. Splenectomy will usually normalize the hematocrit. Hereditary elliptocytosis is a similar disorder associated
with peripheral elliptocytes. It is infrequently associated with
severe hemolysis and usually represents more of a morphologic curiosity
than a clinical problem.

• The following data base supports a diagnosis of HS.

  • Positive family history

  • Splenomegaly

  • History of gallstones

  • Positive autohemolysis test

  • Positive osmotic fragility test

ACUTE HEMOLYSIS IN PATIENTS WHO ARE BLACK OR OF MEDITERRANEAN ANCESTRY

In black and Mediterranean populations the presence of hemolysis
suggests G-6-PD deficiency, thalassemia (p. 14) or a hemoglobinopathy
(p. 56). Clearly G-6-PD deficiency occurs in other than black, Greek
or Italian patients, and such patients may hemolyze for reasons other

than G-6-PD deficiency. However it is worth focusing on the above association, as most patients with G-6-PD hemolysis in this country are black or of Mediterranean ancestry.

Remember:

- 10% of black males in the United States are affected (hemizygotes, sex-linked inheritance).

- 20% of black females are heterozygotes (1% are homozygotes).

- In the black patient G-6-PD deficiency causes only an acute self-limited hemolytic anemia, whereas the Caucasian type of G-6-PD hemolysis is more severe and one may see chronic ongoing compensated or partially compensated hemolysis.

- Hemolysis is precipitated usually by infections (bacterial, viral) or certain drugs (see p. 44) and rarely by severe acidosis.

- Hemolysis is classically intravascular with transitory hemoglobinemia, hemoglobinuria and delayed hemosiderinuria. However, this evidence of intravascular destruction is frequently missed.

Diagnosis

- One sometimes sees a characteristic cell on smear ("bite cell," "blister cell") at the height of the hemolysis (p. 34).

- Screening tests for the enzyme deficiency are not always positive:

  1. Around 30% of heterozygote females have a normal G-6-PD screening test.

  2. Following hemolysis (when the affected cells have been destroyed), the heterozygote (especially with the African type of enzyme deficiency) usually gives a normal screen and may not be diagnosable until G-6-PD-deficient cells accumulate again in significant numbers (several weeks).

  3. In the African type even the hemizygote male may have a normal screen following hemolysis. Although all of his cells are deficient, young cells have significant enzyme levels which drop only as cells age. A male with the Caucasian type of deficiency is usually easily diagnosed even after hemolysis.

- Remember that Heinz body formation is very transitory and requires special staining techniques to visualize. Heinz body identification is not a clinically practical diagnostic test for G-6-PD deficiency hemolysis.

Typical Case

A young, previously healthy black woman presents with typical infectious hepatitis:

. Hct - 19%

. Reticulocytes - 18%

. Peripheral smear - polychromatophilia, "shift cells" and "bite cells"

. Urine hemoglobin is present in the absence of hematuria

. Haptoglobin is saturated

. Several days later the urine sediment stains positively for iron (positive urine hemosiderin test)

. G-6-PD screen normal

. G-6-PD screen 2 months later - positive for G-6-PD deficiency

There is no specific treatment other than avoidance of those drugs known to initiate oxidative hemolysis. Recovery from hemolysis is usually rapid. Rare cases of acute renal failure have been reported. Occasionally transfusion may be necessary. In the African type, patients are protected from repeat hemolysis until cells age and drop their enzyme levels, again becoming susceptible to an oxidative stress.

Common Drugs Implicated in G-6-PD Hemolysis

Sulfonamides
Sulfones
Naphthalene
Primaquine
Nitrofurantoin

REFERENCES

Brain MC: Microangiopathic hemolytic anemia. N Engl J Med 281:833, 1969.
Beutler E: Glucose-6-phosphate dehydrogenase deficiency: diagnosis, clinical and genetic implications. Am J Clin Pathol 47:303, 1967.
Dameshek W: Hypersplenism. Bull NY Acad Med 31:113, 1955.

Hillman RS, Finch CA: Red Cell Manual. Philadelphia, FA Davis, 1978, pp 7-12, 18-19, 40-46.

Jacobson LB, Longstreth GF, Edgington TS: Clinical and immunologic features of transient cold agglutinin hemolytic anemia. Am J Med 54:514, 1973.

Perotta AL, Finch CA: The polychromatophilic erythrocyte. Am J Clin Path 57:471, 1972.

Petz LD: Red cell transfusion problems in immunohematologic disease. Annu Rev Med 33:355-361, 1982.

Pirofsky B: Clinical aspects of autoimmune hemolytic anemia. Semin Hematol 13:251, 1976.

Rosenfeld RE, Jagathambal: Transfusion therapy for autoimmune hemolytic anemia. Semin Hematol 13:311, 1976.

Weed RI: Hereditary spherocytosis. Arch Intern Med 135:1316, 1975.

Worlledge, SM: Immune drug induced hemolytic anemias. Semin Hematol 10:327, 1973.

Chapter 5

Anemia with a Normal MCV and Inappropriately Low Reticulocyte Index

Such anemias are among the most common seen in medicine. Before considering possible etiologies and embarking on a diagnostic workup, make sure:

1. The Hct/Hgb is reproducibly low. Know the normals for your laboratory. In some laboratories an Hct of 34% in a woman is normal. Recognize the variation in normals based on sex, age, and pregnancy (see p. 1).

2. That volume overload is not the etiology (see p. 1).

Table 5.1
Anemia with a Normal MCV and Low Reticulocyte Index

Differential Diagnosis

Renal failure
Anemia of inflammatory disease (anemia of malignancy)
Anemia of hypoendocrine states (hypothyroidism, etc.)
Mild (early) iron deficiency
Combined iron deficiency and megaloblastic anemia
Sideroblastic anemia
Aplastic anemia
Bone marrow infiltration (myelophthisis)
Bleeding or hemolysis plus one of the above

ANEMIA OF RENAL FAILURE

Mechanism

The most important mechanism is decreased marrow erythropoiesis. Decreased marrow red cell production may be secondary to decreased erythropoietin or interference with erythropoietic activity by uremic toxins. In addition there is evidence that excessive parathormone activity may inhibit erythropoiesis in some patients with renal failure and secondary hyperparathyroidism. There is a hemolytic component as well in severe renal insufficiency, but it is usually mild and one for which a normal marrow production would compensate. An occasional patient may develop splenomegaly and severe hemolysis. Be aware that patients on chronic dialysis have other mechanisms for anemia:

- Iron deficiency (bleeding into the coil, phlebotomy, GI bleeding).

- Folate deficiency (folic acid is hemodialyzable).

- Microangiopathic hemolysis (some patients with glomerulopathies, hemolytic uremic syndrome).

Routine Data Base

The RBC morphology is usually normal. One may see occasional spiculated cells ("burr cells"). The occasional patient may have a microangiopathic smear. Polys may be hypersegmented in the absence of folate deficiency. Mild thrombocytopenia (90,000-140,000) is not unusual in severe renal insufficiency. Anemia is unusual if the creatinine is less than 3. The Hct level, even in severe renal failure (dialysis), is extremely variable (low teens with a transfusion requirement to the mid-30s).

Further Data Base

Note the following:

- Commercial erythropoietin assays are not yet reliable.

- Serum ferritin is useful in the diagnosis of iron deficiency accompanying chronic renal failure. However, the lower limit of normal is significantly higher than in patients with normal renal function (see p. 13).

- SI and TIBC are unreliable for making a diagnosis of iron deficiency in these patients.

Treatment

Hemodialysis patients are benefited by the following:

- Leaving the kidneys in place if possible (average Hcts are 4-5% higher).

- Routine androgen administration will increase production and the peripheral Hct (3-5%) in some patients.

.   Supplemental iron and folate administration (common deficiencies).

.   Limiting blood drawing.

.   Peritoneal dialysis patients have higher hematocrits than hemodialysis patients (more effective in removing those toxins which depress erythropoiesis).

.   Splenectomy will benefit the occasional patient with hypersplenism and marked hemolysis.

ANEMIA OF INFLAMMATION (MALIGNANCY)

Clinical Setting

This is one of the most common mechanisms of anemia and is seen in the setting of almost any chronic inflammatory state. This anemia has been best studied in rheumatoid arthritis but may be seen in chronic infections, chronic inflammatory liver disease, chronic inflammatory joint disease other than rheumatoid (inflammatory osteoarthritis, gout, etc.), active collagen vascular disease, etc. The mechanism of anemia seen commonly in cancer patients is similar. In addition to these chronic conditions anemia may also develop during acute infections or inflammation of other types.

Mechanism

The major mechanism is decreased RBC production, although there is also a slight shortening of RBC survival. Decreased production appears to be associated with some decrease in erythropoietic activity as well as abnormal iron kinetics.

Routine Data Base

The RBC morphology is normal. The MCV is usually normal but may be less than 80. This anemia is mild to moderate. This mechanism does not explain an Hct of less than 25%.

Further Data Base

The SI is low and, if the anemia is chronic, the TIBC is low as well. The percent saturation may be as low as 10%. The serum ferritin is normal or elevated, and bone marrow iron stores are normal or increased. As with chronic renal failure, the serum ferritin can be used to diagnose iron deficiency in patients with chronic inflammatory states; however, the lower limit of normal is higher. A number of malignancies are associated with elevated serum ferritin levels (p. 13).

Remember:

- Acute infections (viral, bacterial, etc.) may cause an immediate decrease in marrow production, reticulocytopenia and a drop in the SI. If present for 1-2 weeks, an Hct drop of several percentage points may occur.

- Acute infections (or inflammation of other types (may inhibit the normal bone marrow response to any anemia (bleeding, hemolysis, etc.).

ANEMIA OF HYPOENDOCRINE STATES

Mechanism

The anemia of hypothyroidism (present in 25% of patients) is the best studied; however, anemia also occurs in hypoadrenalism and hypopituitarism. The chief mechanism appears to be decreased production secondary to decreased erythropoietin production probably related to lessened peripheral oxygen requirements. Other mechanisms for anemia are common in patients with hypothyroidism:

1. Pernicious anemia - 10%

2. Iron deficiency (women because of metrorrhagia) - 15%

3. Anemia of hypothyroidism - 25%

Routine Data Base

The anemia is usually mild (Hcts in low 30s). The MCV is normal or high normal. A macrocytic anemia in hypothyroidism (MCV > 100) is usually due to pernicious anemia. The MCV in the anemia of hypothyroidism frequently falls slowly with treatment but is usually not > 100. RBCs on smear appear normal. In up to 30% of patients one may find occasional spiculated cells (morphology similar to the "burr cells" seen in renal disease).

Further Data Base

Studies for B12 deficiency and iron deficiency are appropriate when the routine data base suggests these diagnoses. A high percentage of patients have antibodies to parietal cells and intrinsic factor. Gastric achlorhydria is common.

Treatment

Thyroid replacement results in a slow rise in the hematocrit which may not normalize for many months.

MILD IRON DEFICIENCY

Iron deficiency is discussed in Chapter 2. Remember that the
MCV and peripheral smear RBC morphology may be normal in early, mild
iron deficiency anemia. The serum ferritin and bone marrow iron stain
will be the most helpful diagnostic tests in such cases. Remember
that in very early iron deficiency anemia the serum ferritin may be
in the low normal range at a time when the bone marrow reveals absent
iron stores.

COMBINED IRON DEFICIENCY AND MEGALOBLASTIC ANEMIA

It is not uncommon to see iron deficiency and folate deficiency
occurring together in the alcoholic patient or the patient with severe
inflammatory small bowel disease. Iron deficiency is also occasionally
seen in association with PA.

Routine Data Base

The MCV may be normal, high or low. The smear may show
macroovalocytes as well as small hypochromic cells, but the smear
may be relatively unhelpful in distinguishing combined deficiency
from megaloblastic anemia alone.

Further Data Base

Usual diagnostic tests for iron deficiency and folate/B12
deficiency (p. 11, 20).

SIDEROBLASTIC ANEMIA

Sideroblastic anemia is a syndrome with many different etiologies
associated with the presence of ringed sideroblasts seen on a bone
marrow iron stain.

Sideroblastic Anemia: Differential Diagnosis

Congenital
Acquired

   Primary idiopathic
   Secondary

      Drugs (alcohol, lead, antituberculosis drugs,
         chloramphenicol)
      Collagen vascular disease
      Multiple myeloma
      Marked hemolysis
      Thalassemia

Megaloblastic anemia
Preleukemia and the non lymphocytic acute leukemias

The mechanism has been best worked out in the congenital and drug-induced cases. Inhibition of heme metabolism within the mitochrondria is associated with iron loading of the nucleated RBC mitochrondria which are situated in a perinuclear location, resulting in the morphologic picture seen on iron staining of nucleated RBCs. Alcohol is by far the most common etiology and is frequently seen associated with folate-deficient megaloblastosis. The acquired idiopathic form manifests itself as a refractory anemia seen in elderly patients. Some of these patients progress to develop acute nonlymphocytic leukemia, sometimes after many years.

Routine Data Base

In the congenital and primary idiopathic forms of the disease there is usually marked anisocytosis and poikilocytosis. There is frequently a population of hypochromic, microcytic cells, giving the appearance of two populations of cells. The MCV, however, is usually normal or slightly elevated. It may on occasion be decreased (congenital forms). Coarse stippling (Pappenheimer bodies, p. 5) is almost always present but may require a tedious search to find. The bone marrow picture varies with etiology but usually shows erythroid hyperplasia. Iron stain reveals the presence of ringed sideroblasts (nucleated RBCs staining heavily from iron located in the perinuclear mitochrondria).

Further Data Base

The SI is frequently elevated. The serum ferritin is high. Other data will vary depending on etiology. The primary idiopathic and preleukemic forms of the disease may mimic megaloblastic anemia, but the serum B12 and serum folate levels are normal or elevated and there is no response to B12 or folic acid.

Treatment

Treatment depends on etiology:

- Alcohol - alcohol withdrawal/folic acid administration

- Megaloblastic anemia - folate/B12

- Drug induced - drug withdrawal, chelation treatment for lead

- Primary idiopathic acquired and congenital forms - Pyridoxine in pharmacologic doses (200 mg per day). Occasional cases may respond only to the active metabolite of pyridoxine (pyridoxal-5-phosphate).

APLASTIC ANEMIA

Chronic aplastic anemia will not be described in detail. Severe cases require specialized treatment in a center equipped for bone marrow transplantation. The red cells usually appear normal or demonstrate moderate anisocytosis. The MCV may be normal or slightly elevated. There is a peripheral pancytopenia which may be marked, and the bone marrow is markedly hypocellular. Note that chemotherapy-induced aplasia (Imuran, 6-mercaptopurine, methotrexate, hydroxyurea, 5-fluorouracil, cytosine arbinoside, etc.) frequently results in a macrocytic peripheral RBC population with morphologic changes of a megaloblastic anemia.

ANEMIA ASSOCIATED WITH BONE MARROW INFILTRATION

Marrow infiltration from many different causes is usually associated with a normocytic anemia. When infiltration is extensive, there are frequently classic peripheral blood findings present. These findings, known as leukoerythroblastosis, include:

1. Marked variation in red cell shape, "tear drop" cells being common.

2. Nucleated RBCs.

3. Left shift in the granulocytes with myelocytes being seen on smear.

Apparently the disrupted marrow releases cells early. Red cells inappropriately released, still containing cytoplasmic and nuclear fragments, are distorted during splenic passage to produce the poikilocytosis.

Leukoerythroblastosis (Common Etiologies)

Primary myelofibrosis (Agnogenic myeloid metaplasia)
End-stage polycythemia vera
Metastatic cancer

Breast
Prostate
Oat cell carcinoma of the lung

Acute leukemia (occasionally)
Other hematologic malignancies on occasion (CLL, multiple myeloma, lymphosarcoma).

Leukoerythroblastosis is not a sensitive indicator of bone marrow involvement in metastatic cancer. It is present in fewer than 25%

of cases with a positive bone marrow biopsy for tumor. Anemia is present in most cases with positive bone marrow biopsies.

ANEMIA IN THE ELDERLY

Old age is not an explanation for a significant normocytic anemia. Average hematocrits in patients in their 70s and 80s are only 1-2 percentage points lower than the normal general adult range.

THE PERIPHERAL SMEAR

The peripheral RBC morphology confirms the lack of appropriate bone marrow response in these anemias (no increase in polychromatophilia). Some of these conditions are associated with abnormal and sometimes specific RBC morphologic abnormalities (Table 5.2).

Table 5.2
Help from the Peripheral Smear

Normal RBC Morphology

        Anemia of chronic inflammation (malignancy)
        Chronic renal failure (most patients)
        Hypoendocrine states (most patients)
        Early iron deficiency
        Aplastic anemia

Abnormal RBC Morphology

        Combined iron and folate deficiency
        Sideroblastic anemia
        Leukoerythroblastosis
        Renal failure (some patients)
        Hypothyroidism (some patients)

INDICATIONS FOR A BONE MARROW EXAMINATION

In general the bone marrow offers minimal help in the workup of these anemias and should not be employed routinely (Table 5.3).

Table 5.3
Help from the Bone Marrow

Bone Marrow Not Helpful

    Anemia of chronic disease
    Chronic renal failure
    Hypoendocrine states

Bone Marrow Helpful

    Myelophthisis (need a marrow biopsy)
    Iron deficiency (serum ferritin is cheaper and less
      uncomfortable)
    Combined iron deficiency and megaloblastic anemia
    Sideroblastic anemia
    Aplastic anemia
    Primary marrow malignancy (leukemia, myeloma, etc.)

THE PATIENT WITH A CHRONIC, VERY MILD ANEMIA AND NO OBVIOUS CAUSE

One of the most frustrating problems encountered by the house officer is that of a very mild anemia (e.g., Hct 35 in a woman or 40 in a man) with a normal MCV, normal smear, normal reticulocyte count and no clues as to etiology from the problem list. Consider the following explanations:

1.   Fluid overload

2.   Recent considerable blood loss from phlebotomy during hospitalization, especially in the setting of a febrile illness inhibiting bone marrow response.

3.   Recent inflammatory problem (including viral infection, recent myocardial infarction, etc.)

4.   Remember that 2.5% of a normal population will have a hematocrit lower than the lower limit of normal.

Recommendations:

1.   Consider the differential diagnosis listed earlier in the chapter and the comments above.

2.   If none seem likely or pertinent and the anemia has just been recognized (especially during a recent hospitalization), it is reasonable to follow the Hct for the present in the outpatient setting without further diagnostic workup, but

realizing the presence of an unexplained problem.

3. If it is known that the anemia is relatively recent (e.g., normal Hct 3 months ago), it should be explained. Consider first:

    a. Occult GI bleeding and early iron deficiency anemia.

    b. Anemia of chronic disease/malignancy (has there been recent weight loss, fever, etc?).

4. Think about hypothyroidism. It is frequently unsuspected and not diagnosed until present many months to years.

REFERENCES

Barbour GL: Effect of parathyroidectomy on anemia in chronic renal failure. Arch Intern Med 139:889–891, 1979.

Cartwright GE: The anemia of chronic disorders. Semin Hematol 3:351, 1966.

Camitta BM, Stork R, Thomas ED: Aplastic anemia. N Engl J Med 306:645–652, 712–717, 1982.

Erslev AJ: Management of anemia of chronic renal failure. Clin Nephrol 2:174, 1974.

Fein HG, Rivlin RS: Anemia in thyroid disease. Med Clin North Am 59:1133, 1975.

Hedler ED, Goffinet JA, Ross S, et al: Controlled study of androgen therapy in anemia of patients on maintenance hemodialysis. N Engl J Med 291:1046, 1975.

Kushner JP, Cartwright, GE: Sideroblastic anemia. Adv Intern Med 22:229, 1977.

Lipochitz DA, Cook JD, Finch CA: A clinical evaluation of serum ferritin as an index of iron stores. N Engl J Med 290:1213, 1974.

Thomas FD, Fefer A, Buckner CD, et al: Current status of bone marrow transplantation for aplastic anemia and acute leukemia. Blood 49:671, 1977.

Zappacosta AR, Caro J, Erslev A: Normalization of hematocrit in patients with end stage renal disease on continuous ambulatory peritoneal dialysis. Am J Med 72:53–57, 1982.

Chapter 6

Hemoglobin S and Hemoglobin C Disorders

Congenital disorders associated with abnormal globin chains may cause several different clinical syndromes:

- Hemolysis (unstable hemoglobins, e.g., Hgb Zurich)

- Erythrocytosis (increased Hgb O_2 affinity, e.g., Hgb Chesapeake)

- Cyanosis (e.g., Hgb Kansas and Hgb Seattle)

The above syndromes are quite rare in comparison with hemoglobin S and hemoglobin C disorders.

HEMOGLOBIN S

- A β chain mutation resulting in rigid elongated tactoids which distort red cell shape and increase red cell rigidity. Clumps of sickled cells lead to tissue ischemia and infarction.

- 10% of the black population in the United States are heterozygous for Hgb S (Hgb AS).

- The gene is also present to a lesser extent in Greeks, Italians, Arabians and Asian Indians.

- The mutation affords protection from endemic malaria.

Sickle Cell Trait (Hgb AS)

- For the most part sickle trait individuals are completely well, although a large number of rare clinical problems have been associated with the sickle cell trait defect. Those for which there are reasonable data to support a cause-effect relationship are:

1. Splenic infarction at high altitudes.
2. Episodic hematuria.

56

3. Increased incidence of bacteriuria including bacteriuria
    and pyelonephritis in pregnancy.

4. Hyposthenuria.

There are many other anecdotal associations which are much less
well documented.

*   The peripheral smear is normal. Sickling is seen only on a sickle
    cell prep (deoxygenated blood).

*   Hemoglobin electrophoresis reveals around 40% Hgb S and the rest
    Hgb A, with a small amount of Hgb F and Hgb A2.

*   Once identified, sickle cell trait individuals should receive:

    1. Genetic counseling:

        a. Information as to the incidence of Hgb S gene.

        b. A couple, both heterozygous for Hgb S, have a 25% chance
            of having a child with sickle cell anemia.

    2. Assurance that they are essentially clinically normal and
        that complications from their carrying the sickle cell gene
        are extremely rare.

    3. Education about the nature of the sickling defect.

Sickle Cell Anemia (Hgb SS)

Hemoglobin SS disease exists in approximately 0.25% of the black
population in the United States. Clinical sequelae of this severe
disease differ depending on whether one sees primarily a pediatric
or adult population. The pediatrician primarily sees infectious complications related to decreased pneumococcal opsonin formation, decreased
RES phagocytosis and possible increased bacterial load from GI ischemia.
Pneumococcal and Haemophilus infections predominate. Salmonella osteomyelitis is common as well. The physician caring for adults primarily
sees organ dysfunction complications, the result of repeated ischemic
events in various body organs. Both commonly see painful sickle cell
crises.

General Laboratory Findings

Anemia. Frequently slightly macrocytic because of the reticulo-
    cytosis. Hct ranges from high teens to low 30s. The mechanism
    is primarily hemolytic, and a chronic indirect hyperbilirubinemia
    is common.

Leukocytosis. There may be a chronic neutrophilia, and WBC counts
    may rise to 30,000-40,000 per μl with pain crises.

Thrombocytosis. Usually mild. May be greater than 1,000,000 per μl.

Reticulocytosis.

Peripheral smear. Markedly distorted red cell shapes with classic sickled erythrocytes being evident on a routine smear. Poly-chromatophilia is prominent. Howell-Jolley bodies and Pappenheimer bodies are commonly seen as features of autosplenectomy from sickling (usually occurring before age 10). Target cells are frequent (most prominent in SC disease).

Hgb electrophoresis. Reveals only Hgb S with a variable amount of Hgb F (no Hgb A).

Effect on various organ systems

Bone

There are a number of clinical and radiologic features commonly seen in sickle cell bone disease:

- Widened medullary spaces seen in the proximal long bones and skull due to the marked compensatory bone marrow expansion.

- "Codfish" spine: Central circumscribed areas of depression in the vertebral end plates.

- Ischemia and infarction leading to changes which mimic those of osteomyelitis (periosteal reaction, osteosclerosis, etc.). Osteomyelitis is common as well.

- Dactylitis (hand-foot syndrome). Acute swelling of hands and feet seen in the infant.

- Aseptic necrosis of the femoral (and rarely humoral) head (more common in Hgb SC disease).

- Bone marrow necrosis with sometimes bone marrow emboliz-ation.

- Growth is inhibited, so that children are short but puberty is delayed and many adult sickle cell patients are tall with long thin extremities.

Spleen

- Splenomegaly disappears usually by age 8 due to repeated infarctions. This autosplenectomy state contributes to the tendency to infection and causes some of the peripheral blood changes noted above. A syndrome known as <u>splenic sequestration crisis</u> occurs in infants due to massive splenic pooling of red cells. It is frequently fatal.

Liver and Gallbladder

- Hepatomegaly may occur with crises. Abnormal pain crises mimic acute cholecystitis or other abdominal catastrophes.

- Intrahepatic cholestasis secondary to sickling in the sinusoids may occur, resulting in massive hyperbilirubinemia (combination of hemolysis and hepatic dysfunction), with bilirubin levels sometimes greater than 100 mg%.

- Differentiation of the above syndromes from cholecystitis is difficult (50% of adult sickle cell patients have gallstones, mostly radio-opaque bilirubin stones). Indications for cholecystectomy are not clear-cut. Many physicians recommend elective cholecystectomy in sickle cell patients with gallstones who have had abdominal episodes consistent with acute cholecystitis.

Cardiovascular

Patients develop cardiomegaly from chronic anemia and repetitive microinfarctions. Murmurs are frequent and may suggest rheumatic or congenital heart disease.

Pulmonary

Deep venous thrombosis and pulmonary embolism are seen. Pulmonary thrombosis in situ occurs and may be difficult to distinguish from pneumonia. Pulmonary thrombosis/embolism may be extensive and recurrent and lead with time to pulmonary hypertension and right heart failure.

Central Nervous System

Vascular accidents are common, including cerebral infarction, hematomas and subdural and subarachnoid hemorrhage. Seizure disorders are seen frequently.

Leg Ulcers

Up to 75% of patients with SS disease develop leg ulcerations at some time during their lives, and for many the problem is chronic. The following are characteristic features:

- Usually seen on the medial side of the leg above the ankle.

- Typically presents a punched-out appearance and may be quite large.

.   Thought to be due to ischemia in an area where venous pressure is high.

Eye

Sickle cell patients, including patients with SC and S-thalassemia disease, are prone to a serious retinopathy which may lead to blindness and which may be preventable. The following pathophysiologic sequence occurs:

1.   Retinal capillary plugging by sickled cells.

2.   Secondary neovascularization (arborization) resulting in fragile vascular connections between arterioles and venules. They may be seen at the periphery of the retinas and look like a primitive marine animal called a sea fan.

3.   Vitreous hemorrhage secondary to leak in one of these defective vessels.

4.   Retinal detachment as the vitreous hemorrhage scars and retracts.

The above sequence can be interrupted prior to the vitreous hemorrhage by photocoagulation of the abnormal new vessels. Every patient with SS, SC and S-thalassemia disease should have a yearly evaluation by an ophthalmologist with experience in these techniques.

Kidney

SS (SA, SC, S-thal) patients have hyposthenuria and may develop episodes of severe unilateral hematuria secondary to ischemia of the renal medulla. In addition to renal tubular dysfunction, immune complex glomerular disease is sometimes seen.

OTHER SYNDROMES

SC Disease

Milder than SS disease usually. Smear reveals many target cells common with all C hemoglobinopathies. The Hgb electrophoresis reveals about equal levels of Hgb C and Hgb S. The spleen may be palpable.

S-thalassemia Disease

Milder than SS usually. The MCV is usually low. Target cells may be prominent on smear. The spleen may be palpable. In S-β thalassemia, Hgb electrophoresis reveals a pattern of 70-80% S with small amounts of Hgb A and F. In patients with SS disease and α-thalassemia there is frequently a lower MCV, increased level of Hgb F and milder clinical disease, depending on the number and pattern of defective globin genes. The marked variability in severity in patients with SS disease is at least partially explained by this protective effect of concomitant -thalassemia.

C-Trait Disease (Hgb AC)

Usually clinically normal without anemia. The smear reveals large numbers of target cells.

Hgb CC Disease

A mild disease associated with a slight anemia, splenomegaly and occasional mild pain (arthralgia). Infections may be seen, including Salmonella osteomyelitis. The smear reveals target cells and misshapen spherocytes (common in all the C hemoglobinopathies).

TREATMENT

Pain (Thrombotic) Crisis

Pain may involve any area of the body, but commonly involves long bones, the back and the abdomen. The pain is frequently severe, requiring parenteral narcotics. Crises may last a few hours to days and even, rarely, several weeks. The patient may have fever (occasionally to 103°) and an increase in the usual neutrophilia, making differentiation from infection difficult. There is no specific therapy. Hospitalization with appropriate narcotics for pain control is frequently necessary. There are no data to show that nasal oxygen is helpful in the absence of severe hypoxia. It is reasonable to maintain good hydration. The most important medical issue is to rule out infection. It is important that the patient be tapered off of narcotics before discharge, as iatrogenic addiction does occur.

Infection

As mentioned, these patients (especially children) are very prone to infections (pneumococcal, Haemophilus, Salmonella), and patients should be encouraged to see their physicians early for any febrile illness. Because of the sickle cell patient's difficulty with handling penumococcal infections, it is recommended that he or she be immunized with pneumococcal vaccine.

Hemolytic Crisis

Such crises are rare. In adults a hematocrit drop occurring in the setting of a pain crisis should make the physician suspect infection. Remember that infection decreases marrow red cell production, resulting in a rapid hematocrit drop in a patient with severe chronic hemolytic anemia.

Aplastic Crisis

Decreased marrow production results in a dramatic hematocrit drop in these patients. Infection is the most common etiology. Folic acid deficiency may develop because of the patient's increased requirements (marked erythroid hyperplasia). All sickle cell patients should be maintained on supplemental folic acid (1 mg per day).

Thrombosis/Embolization

Sickle cell patients with deep vein thrombosis or pulmonary embolism should be anticoagulated as with any other patient. Pulmonary thrombosis in situ may develop which may be difficult to distinguish from pneumonia in a febrile patient with leukocytosis.

Leg Ulcers

Ulcers, when large, are particularly refractory to treatment. Skin grafting is helpful in only a minority of patients and frequently does not seem worth the time and discomfort involved. Local measures to keep the ulcer clean, frequent elevation, surgical stockings or wraps are all useful. Frequently healing occurs over months only to recur again a few months or years later.

Hematuria

Not uncommon in patients with AS Hgb as well as SS, SC and S-thalassemia. It is thought to be due to medullary ischemia due to the tendency of cells to sickle when subjected to the hypertonic milieu of the renal medulla. Bleeding may occur for days to weeks. Maintaining a high urine flow is usually successful in stopping the hematuria.

Priapism

Priapism is common in SS and SC disease and usually results in permanent impotence once resolved. If seen within the first few hours of onset, urologic intervention may be attempted, but it is not clear that operative intervention is helpful in preventing impotence. Urologic prostheses, once the impotence has occurred, are frequently quite helpful.

PREVENTIVE MEDICINE RECOMMENDATIONS

1. The sickle cell patient has a lifelong chronic illness with frequent and recurrent use of the medical care system. He or she needs:

a. One personal physician.

b. Access to a physician 24 hours a day.

c. A workable system to obtain emergency care 24 hours a day.

2. Daily folic acid (1 mg per day).

3. Rapid medical evaluation for the development of fever/chills.

4. Pneumococcal vaccine.

5. Analgesics. Narcotic addiction does occur. In general, the sickle cell patient should probably not be given oral narcotics for use at home during a pain crisis except in the following situation:

> There is one personal physician who knows the patient and knows that he or she is the only physician writing narcotic prescriptions for the patient. In this situation, with a patient with frequent pain crises, it is not unreasonable to allow the patient a few (10 or 15) codeine or Demerol tablets to be used early during a pain attack in the hope of preventing the necessity for an emergency room visit and hospitalization. Be careful: Iatrogenic addiction does occur.

6. Because of the common presence of heart murmurs which mimic rheumatic valvular disease, it is frequently difficult in the sickle cell patient to rule out the latter. Prophylactic antibiotics with invasive procedures (dental work, etc.) in such patients are reasonable.

7. Transfusions and exchange transfusion therapy. In general, transfusions should be avoided because of the hazard of iron overload. However, with the recent advent of more effective methods of iron chelation (intravenous/subcutaneous infusions of desferrioxamine), transfusions in the future may be utilized more often. Exchange transfusion can probably shorten pain crises and may be useful prior to general anesthesia to decrease the chance of hypoxemia-induced sickling. Chronic hypertransfusion can decrease the number of crises in patients with marked incapacity from chronic recurrent episodes of pain. However, the clinical price of chronic transfusion therapy is so high that most experts are reluctant to advocate such therapy. Perhaps iron chelation therapy in the future may decrease the hazards.

8. Pharmacologic attempts to increase hemoglobin F production hold considerable interest (reported recently in patients with thalassemia and sickle cell disease with treatment with 5-Azacytidine). Attempts to decrease red cell hemoglobin concentration and thus sickling by treatment with vasopressin are also interesting but

probably not practical for chronic therapy.

REFERENCES

Abramson H, Bertles JF, Wethers DL eds: Sickle Cell Disease. St. Louis, CV Mosby, 1973.

Charache S: Treatment of sickle cell anemia. Annu Rev Med 32:195–206, 1981.

Hanosh SM, Rucknagel DL: Clinical implications of recent advances in hemoglobin disorders. Med Clin North Am 64:775–800, 1980.

Higgs DR, et al: The interaction of alpha-thalassemia and homozygous sickle-cell disease. N Engl J Med 306:1441–1446, 1982.

Sang T: Pathology of Sickle Cell Disease. Springfield, IL, Charles C. Thomas, 1971.

Sears DA: The morbidity of sickle-cell trait. Am J Med 64:1021–1036, 1978.

Sergeant, GR: The Clinical Features of Sickle Cell Disease. Amsterdam, North-Holland, 1974.

Chapter 7

Bleeding Disorders:
Approach to Diagnosis

<u>DIAGNOSTIC APPROACH TO BLEEDING</u>

When faced with a bleeding patient or a history of untoward bleeding, the clinician should initially try to answer the following clinical questions:

<u>1.   IS THE BLEEDING FROM MORE THAN ONE SITE?</u>

Bleeding from only one site is usually not due to a bleeding diathesis. Beware of the untied bleeder in the operative wound or the recurrent unilateral nosebleed.

<u>2.   IS THE BLEEDING PROBLEM LIFELONG OR OF RECENT ONSET?</u>

Hereditary bleeding problems are usually easily identified by a history of lifelong bleeding. A family history of bleeding may suggest a pattern of inheritance. However, be wary of the general statement, "I've always been a free bleeder." Apply much greater weight to objective data. For example:

a.   Untoward bleeding with surgery (e.g., tonsillectomy, tooth extraction) especially if <u>transfusions</u> were necessary

b.   Bleeding requiring <u>hospitalization</u> or return to the dentist for control of delayed bleeding

<u>3.   DOES THE PATTERN OF BLEEDING SUGGEST A CLOTTING PROBLEM OR A "HEMOSTATIC PLUG" FORMATION PROBLEM?</u>

a.   Clotting problems (for example, hemophilia)

(1)   Bleeding from large vessels, not capillaries

(2)   Hemarthrosis, large hematomas, large ecchymosis, extensive bleeding with trauma

b.   "Hemostatic plug" (platelet) problems?

  (1)   Small vessel (capillary) bleeding - petechiae

  (2)   Mucous membrane bleeding (nose, gums, GI tract)

  (3)   "Ooze" rather than a "gush"

c.   Some bleeding diatheses are associated with both a clotting and
     a hemostatic plug formation problem (see Chapter 9).

<u>ROUTINE LABORATORY DATA BASE</u>

     The following tests are available and used as screening tests
in most hospitals and represent reasonable and inexpensive baseline
data in the evaluation of all patients with a suspected bleeding diathesis.

  1.   Prothrombin time (PT)

  2.   Activated partial thromboplastin time (aPTT)

  3.   Thrombin time (TT)

  4.   Peripheral smear

  5.   Platelet count (if a smear suggests a decreased or markedly
       increased platelet count).

     The above tests utilizing the widely employed Vacutainer system
require one citrate tube (PT, aPTT, TT), one EDTA tube (platelet count)
and a fingerstick peripheral smear (see p. 70). Beware of the following
pitfalls in obtaining the routine data.

  1.   Citrate tubes usually contain 0.5 cc of anticoagulant to
       which 4.5 cc of blood should be added. This ratio is important.
       Incomplete filling of the tube (e.g., partial loss of vacuum)
       may result in spurious results, especially of the aPTT.

  2.   Coagulation tests should be conducted promptly following
       drawing of blood. The aPTT in particular may be spuriously
       prolonged by delay in assay. The following times are guidelines.

       a.   Room temperature storage - assay within 2 hours.

       b. $4^{o}C$ storage - assay within 12 hours.

  3.   If the aPTT assay cannot be done for 12 hours or more, anti-
       coagulated blood may be spun and the plasma frozen for assay
       later.

  4.   Platelet counts may be conducted after sitting at 4° for
       up to 24 hours. The platelet count may be spuriously increased
       in patients with very high WBC counts (leukemia) or severe

RBC poikilocytosis.

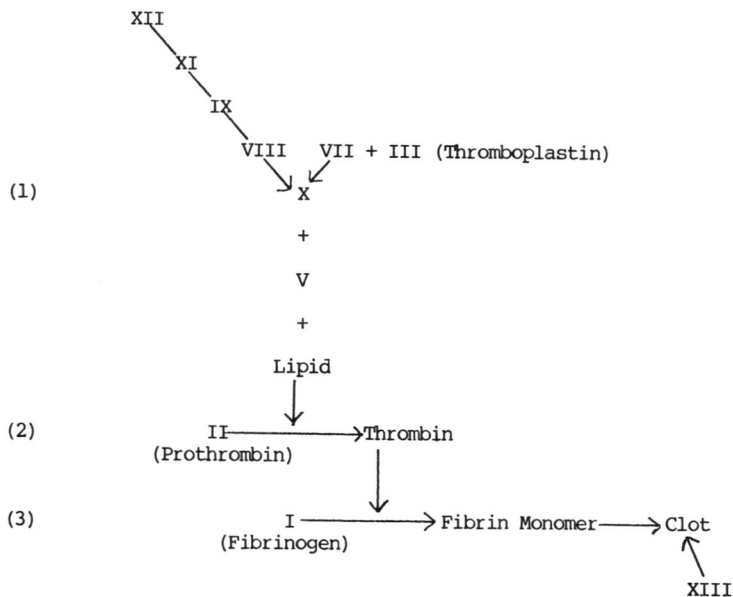

**Figure 7.1
The Coagulation Scheme**

The clotting process involves the activation in cascade fashion of a number of circulating coagulation factors designated by roman numerals in Figure 7.1. Initiation of clotting in vivo usually occurs by one of two methods:

1. The activation of Factor VII by tissue thromboplastin (Factor III) exposed when vessel is disrupted (extrinsic system), or

2. The activation of Factor XII by various means (altered blood vessel surface, endotoxin, complement, kinins, etc.) with the subsequent cascade activation of other coagulation factors "downstream" (intrinsic system).

Activation of Factor X is the common meeting point of both systems. Activated X in the presence of Factor V plus lipid (provided by platelets in vivo) results in the subsequent conversion of prothrombin (Factor II) to thrombin. Thrombin cleaves fibrinogen, the resulting fibrin monomer polymerizes to form a clot which is stabilized by Factor XIII. Ca^{++} is necessary in a number of steps of coagulation (as is platelet lipid). Blood is anticoagulated in vivo by the binding of CA^{++} (usually by citrate).

INDIVIDUAL COAGULATION TESTS

1. Prothrombin Time (PT)

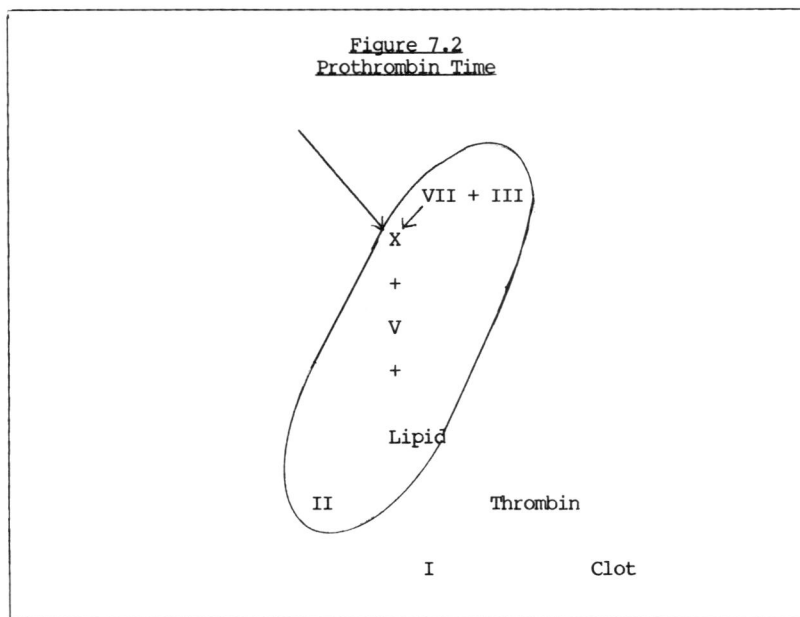

Figure 7.2
Prothrombin Time

The PT measures primarily Factors II, VII, V, and X (circled in Fig. 7.2). Calcium plus tissue thromboplastin (III) is added to citrated plasma, and the time to clot formation is measured (11-13 seconds in most systems). Remember, the presence of anti-thrombins (e.g., heparin) or abnormalities in the third stage of coagulation (fibrin generation) will also affect the PT since the formation of a clot is the endpoint of the test. Note that platelet lipid is not measured by the PT as it is a component of Factor III which is added.

2. Partial Thromboplastin Time (PTT)

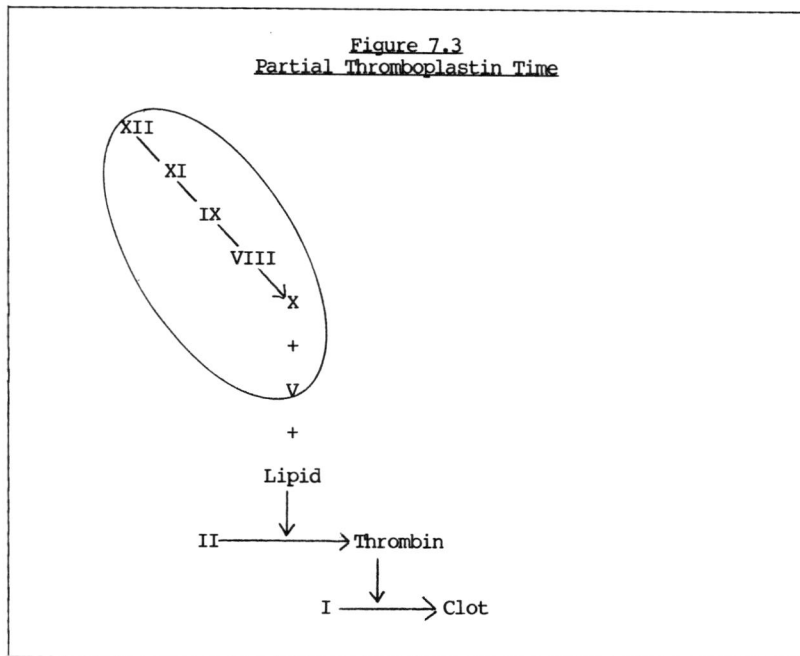

Figure 7.3
Partial Thromboplastin Time

The PTT measures primarily Factors XII, XI, IX, VIII, X and V. Calcium plus lipid is added, and the time to clot formation is measured (usually 25-35 seconds in the activated PTT system). The lipid added is incapable of activating Factor VII but provides the lipid needed in several other steps of coagulation (provided in vivo by platelets). In addition, most PTT systems now utilize an activator of Factor XII (e.g., kaolin) to eliminate the variable of glass activation of XII and to shorten the time of the test (aPTT). As with the PT, remember that subsequent problems in the second and third stages of coagulation will also affect the PT, since the formation of a clot is the endpoint of the test.

3.   Thrombin Time (TT)

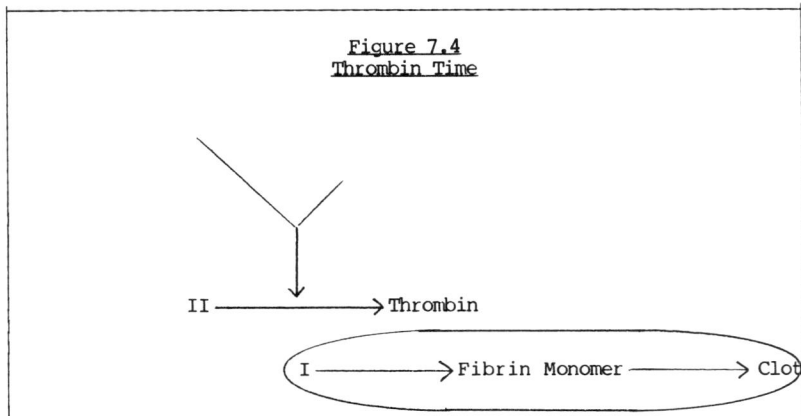

Figure 7.4
Thrombin Time

II ——————————> Thrombin

I ——————————> Fibrin Monomer ——————————> Clot

The TT measures only the third stage of coagulation. Thrombin and Ca^{++} are added, and the time is measured to form a clot. The first and second stages of coagulation are, therefore, bypassed. The TT may be abnormal in the presence of antithrombins (e.g., heparin), with qualitative and quantitative abnormalities of Factor I (fibrinogen) and when there is a problem with fibrin polymerization.

Platelet Function

Platelets function to plug small holes in blood vessels. Initially small numbers of platelets adhere to exposed collagen in the wall of a damaged vessel. Platelets release ADP, which causes large masses of platelets to aggregate ("hemostatic plug" formation) and subsequently release lipid necessary for clot formation. Finally, platelets strengthen the formed clot through clot retraction. In vitro tests of platelet function require sophisticated equipment and are not part of the routine data base in the evaluation of a bleeding diathesis (see p. 82). The bleeding time is generally not part of the initial routine evaluation of a bleeding diathesis (described p. 82) but is indicated when bleeding pattern suggests a hemostatic plug defect and there is no significant decrease in platelet count.

Peripheral Smear and Platelet Count

The peripheral smear may reveal thrombocytopenia or, rarely, marked thrombocytosis in patients with a bleeding diathesis (p. 85). In addition, platelet morphology on occasion may be useful (p. 73).

Remember that the smear should be fingerstick, as anticoagulant distorts platelet morphology (swollen, large).

Platelets may distribute unevenly on a fingerstick smear, so that a "bottle smear" (a smear made from anticoagulated blood) may be better for assessing platelet numbers (the one thing for which a bottle smear is helpful). Red cell morphology may also be helpful, as in DIC where fragmented red cells (schistocytes, p. 33) may be seen on smear. White cell morphology may also be helpful, as when polys reveal the changes associated with sepsis (p. 125) in a patient with DIC.

It is difficult to describe the technique of estimating the platelet count from the peripheral smear, but technicians with considerable experience may become quite good at it. The following generalizations may be useful.

1. Platelets are normally present in clumps on smear.

2. Clumps disappear and only single platelets are seen as the count drops to the 100,000 per ul range and below.

3. Normally several platelets, some in clumps, are seen in each oil emersion field.

4. Be aware on a fingerstick smear that platelets may be unequally distributed, located primarily along the sides of the smear.

REFERENCE

Zieve PD, Levin J: Disorders of Hemostasis. Philadelphia, WB Saunders, 1976.

Chapter 8

Disorders of Platelets

As described in Chapter 6, platelets form the major line of defense against bleeding from small holes in small vessels. Their "hemostatic plug" function requires adequate platelet numbers as well as normal platelet function.

Platelets made in the bone marrow normally circulate for approximately 10 days before removal from the circulation. Young platelets are more functional than old platelets and appear larger on a peripheral smear.

Table 8.1
Thrombocytopenia: Differential Diagnosis

Decreased Survival, Sequestration

        Hypersplenism
        TTP/hemolytic uremic syndrome
        DIC
        Sepsis
        Immune thrombocytopenia

Decreased Production

        Myelophthisis
        Primary bone marrow disorders
        Infection
        Drugs (marrow depressant)

Ineffective Production

        Megaloblastic processes

The normal platelet count, with use of automatic counters, is in the range of 150,000 to 350,000 per μl. There are technical problems which may yield erroneously low counts. A platelet count, or at least an estimation of platelet numbers on a peripheral smear, is part of the routine data base obtained on any patient with a suspected bleeding diathesis. The routine data obtained in patients with thrombocytopenia include the following:

Routine Data Base

- Platelet count.

- Examination of platelet morphology on a **fingerstick** peripheral smear.

- Bone Marrow examination (not always necessary).

- History and physical examination with review of the problem list for likely etiologies of thrombocytopenia.

Etiologic Hints from the Routine Data Base

1. **Severe thrombocytopenia** (platelet counts less than 10,000) — Think of:

   Immune thrombocytopenia.
   Severe aplastic anemia (including drug-induced bone marrow depression).
   Acute leukemia.

2. **Peripheral smear platelet morphology** — Remember:

   - **Young** platelets are large and frequently elongated. In severe thrombocytopenia the presence of such platelets suggests a destructive/sequestration mechanism (e.g., immune thrombocytopenia).

   - **Old** platelets are small. A predominance of small platelets on a smear in **severe** thrombocytopenia suggests a production mechanism (e.g., aplastic anemia).

3. **Bone marrow megakaryocytes**

   a. Increased in destructive thrombocytopenia.

   b. Decreased in productive thrombocytopenia.

   c. Frequently increased in ineffective megakaryopoiesis (e.g., in megaloblastic processes). Other bone marrow findings usually help to distinguish between a and c.

On the basis of the above considerations, the physician should attempt to classify the basic mechanism of the thrombocytopenia:

BASIC MECHANISM

1. Shortened platelet survival or increased peripheral sequestration.

2. Decreased production.

3. Ineffective production.

Table 8.2
Thrombocytopenia: Routine Data Base

Mechanism	Platelet Size	Megakaryocyte Numbers
Decreased survival	Large	Increased
Decreased production	Small	Decreased
Ineffective production	Variable	Normal or increased

Shortened Platelet Survival or Increased Sequestration
(Megakaryocytic Thrombocytopenia)

Normally, platelets survive for around 10 days once released into the circulation. Approximately 30% of the circulating platelets are sequestered at any one time in the spleen. Table 8.3 lists disorders which are associated with decreased survival and/or increased splenic sequestration:

Routine Data Base

- The platelet count may be mildly or severely decreased. When it is less than 20,000, suspect immune thrombocytopenia.

- Platelet morphology on a fingerstick smear reveals large, frequently elongated platelets (young platelets are large).

- The bone marrow reveals increased numbers of megakaryocytes.

Table 8.3
Megakaryocytic Thrombocytopenia: Differential Diagnosis

> Hypersplenism
> TTP/hemolytic uremic syndrome
> DIC
> Infection
> Immune thrombocytopenia

1. **Hypersplenism**

Thrombocytopenia may occur with splenomegaly of almost any etiology, although sometimes it is not present even with massive splenic enlargement. Often leukopenia is present as well. Significant anemia is less frequent.

Treatment

Thrombocytopenia is rarely severe enough to require splenectomy in hypersplenism. Patients with leukemic reticuloendotheliosis and pancytopenia benefit from splenectomy, as occasionally do patients with CLL, lymphosarcomas and myeloproliferative diseases.

2. **Thrombotic Thrombocytopenic Purpura (TTP)/Hemolytic Uremic (HU) Syndromes**

These syndromes are associated with microangiopathic hemolysis with schistocytes (p. 40) seen on peripheral smear. Fever and neurologic dysfunction are common. Renal failure is prominent in the hemolytic uremic syndrome. Etiology is obscure and treatment anecdotal. Plasma transfusion, plasmapheresis (or whole blood exchange) and antiplatelet aggregation therapy (ASA, dipyridamole) are currently favored.

3. **DIC**

Thrombocytopenia is essentially always present in acute DIC, but the bone marrow may be able to compensate completely (platelet count normal) for the shortened platelet survival when DIC is chronic (see p. 94). Platelets return to normal slowly (over days) once the cause for DIC is corrected.

4. **Sepsis**

Patients with septicemia, especially Gram-negative sepsis, may have thrombocytopenia in the absence of other evidence for DIC. Endotoxin will cause platelet sequestration in the capillary circulation. Infections (including viral

infections) may decrease platelet production as well. Treatment
is directed at the underlying infection, not the thrombocytopenia
per se.

5.   Immune Thrombocytopenia

Table 8.4
Immune Thrombocytopenia: Differential Diagnosis

Primary (ITP)
Secondary

    Acute viral infections
    Drugs (quinine, quinidine, sulfonamide derivatives)
    Collagen vascular disorders (SLE)
    Lymphoproliferative disorders
    Graves disease
    Immunodeficiency states

    Antibody-mediated thrombocytopenia occurs in the conditions
listed in Table 8.4. Proof of antibody mechanism in individual
cases is difficult. In vitro testing for platelet-associated
IgG is widely available and can be helpful to confirm an
immunologic mechanism. Although reasonably sensitive, the
test suffers from a lack of specificity. Immune thrombocytopenia
is frequently severe (commonly less than 10,000). Acute
immune thrombocytopenia is frequently drug induced and rapidly
clears with drug withdrawal.

Table 8.5
Some Drugs Implicated in Acute Immune Thrombocytopenia

    Quinine (frequently used to cut heroin)
    Quinidine
    Sulfonamides
    Rifampin
    Thiazide diuretics
    Furosemide
    Chlorthalidone
    Dilantin
    Gold salts
    Heparin

Treatment

Acute immune thrombocytopenia usually requires no specific treatment other than discontinuation of drugs (if implicated). Platelet counts usually return to normal in a few days. If the thrombocytopenia is severe (less than 10,000) or there is clinical bleeding (marked petechiae, nosebleeds, etc.), many physicians recommend short course of steroids (e.g., 40-60 mg of prednisone in divided doses with rapid tapering over 10 days to 3 weeks once counts return).

Chronic idiopathic immune thrombocytopenia (ITP, also designated autoimmune thrombocytopenic purpura, ATP) is usually initially treated with steroids (e.g., 40-100 mg of prednisone per day in divided doses). Response is seen within 2-3 weeks in 60-70% of patients. Once the platelet count rises to the 100,000 range, tapering of the prednisone may begin. A drop in prednisone to 40 mg per day (10 mg q6h) can usually be accomplished immediately. Subsequent tapering is usually at a rate of around 5 mg per week. Some patients can be tapered completely off of steroids without a drop in platelet count. Others will require some ongoing dose of steroid to maintain an adequate platelet count. Splenectomy is usually considered when:

1. The initial steroid treatment (3 weeks) does not significantly elevate the platelet count.

2. An unacceptable steroid dose (15 mg of prednisone per day or greater) is required to maintain the platelet count at greater than 50,000.

3. CNS bleeding occurs. Many feel emergency splenectomy is the treatment of choice for this life-threatening rare complication of severe immune thrombocytopenia. The overall response rate is higher, and, most importantly, the average time to response is shorter than with steroid treatment.

Presently the indications for splenectomy are not clearcut. A syndrome of overwhelming pneumococcal (or Haemophilus) sepsis is seen rarely in adults postsplenectomy (very common in young children, in whom splenectomy is contraindicated under the age of 6). The recognition of this rare but usually fatal syndrome has made many hematologists slower to recommend splenectomy for their patients. Severe bleeding in ITP is unusual even with chronic severe thrombocytopenia.

Chronic secondary immune thrombocytopenia is treated

much like ITP but with more emphasis placed on treatment of the underlying disease. Patients with underlying lymphoproliferative disorders frequently have a refractory thrombocytopenia until the underlying disease is controlled.

Immunosuppression therapy. There are rare patients with very low platelet counts who do not respond to steroids or splenectomy. There are occasional responses in such patients with a number of agents known to have immunosuppressant activity (Imuran, Cytoxan, vincristine, vinblastine, colchicine).

Decreased Platelet Production
(Amegakaryocytic Thrombocytopenia)

Routine Data Base

- The platelet count may be mildly or severely depressed.

- The fingerstick peripheral smear usually reveals small isolated platelets, reflecting the increased average age of the circulating platelets (old platelets are small).

- The bone marrow reveals decreased or absent megakaryocytes and may be diagnostic of a specific etiology (e.g., aplastic anemia, acute leukemia).

Table 8.6
Amegakaryocytic Thrombocytopenia: Differential Diagnosis

Myelophthisis
Primary bone marrow disorders
Infection
Drugs

---

1. Myelophthisis

Actually, solid tumors metastatic to the bone marrow usually do not result in thrombocytopenia. However, when marrow metastases are extensive, as in breast or prostate cancer, platelet counts may fall late in the course of the illness. Infiltrative marrow disease (e.g., Gaucher's disease) result in thrombocytopenia more because of hypersplenism than because of decreased production. Thrombocytopenia by this mechanism is usually seen only with extensive marrow involvement, and leukoerythroblastosis is common on smear (p. 52). Thrombocytopenia is usually not severe, and treatment is directed toward the underlying disorder.

2. Primary Bone Marrow Disorders

Chronic myeloproliferative disease (polycythemia vera, primary thrombocythemia, chronic granulocytic leukemia) usually cause thrombocytosis, not thrombocytopenia. Patients with primary myelofibrosis may have normal platelet numbers, thrombocytopenia or thrombocytosis. Acute leukemias, chronic lymphocytic leukemia, multiple myeloma and leukemic reticuloendotheliosis may all be associated with a production amegakaryocytic thrombocytopenia. Aplastic anemia is frequently associated with severe production thrombocytopenia (see p. 51).

Treatment

It is this group of amegakaryocytic thrombocytopenias in which severe thrombocytopenia with bleeding may occur. In the patient with acute leukemia undergoing chemotherapy, platelet transfusions are given routinely when platelet counts fall to the range of 30,000 or less (see p. 52). Of special importance is the patient with severe aplastic anemia. Bone marrow transplantation has become the treatment of choice for many of these patients. Optimally they should be evaluated early by a center specializing in bone marrow transplantation before transfusions induce sensitization to HLA antigens which may jeopardize a successful transplant.

3. Infection

Viral infections commonly result in decreased platelet production. Mild thrombocytopenias are common (especially in children) with many viral illnesses. Occasionally thrombocytopenia is due to peripheral destruction from antibody as well. Bacterial infections may also result in decreased production as well as increased sequestration with sepsis.

4. Drugs

Thiazides and alcohol are perhaps the most common drug causes of production thrombocytopenia. Chronic high intake of alcohol may cause a severe thrombocytopenia with return to normal within 7-10 days after withdrawal. Other mechanisms of thrombocytopenia in the alcoholic include folic acid deficiency and hypersplenism secondary to liver disease. Thiazides may rarely be associated with an antibody-mediated destructive thrombocytopenia. More commonly one sees a mild production thrombocytopenia, which usually returns to normal rapidly once the drug is discontinued. Other agents have occasionally been implicated as the etiology of isolated amegakaryocytic thrombocytopenia.

Other drug-induced production thrombocytopenias are usually associated with leukopenia and anemia as well (cancer chemotherapeutic agents, immunosuppressive agents, gold and the rare idiosyncratic reactions to chloramphenicol, butazolidin, etc.).

Ineffective Platelet Production

In conditions associated with ineffective megakaryopoiesis, megakaryocytes are present in the bone marrow but platelet production
is defective. The most common example is megaloblastic anemia due
to folate or B12 deficiency and drug-induced megaloblastosis. In
these disorders there is classically a pancytopenia with a markedly
hypercellular, but qualitatively abnormal, bone marrow. Defective
cell production leads to intramarrow destruction of precursor cells
and defective delivery of platelets, white cells and red cells to
the periphery. Other conditions with hypercellularity and ineffective
platelet production include: (1) some cases of sideroblastic anemia,
(2) preleukemia, and (3) paroxysmal nocturnal hemoglobinuria.

Hazards of Invasive Procedures in Patients
with Thrombocytopenia

It is difficult to make generalizations about the relative hazards
of biopsies and other invasive procedures in patients who are thrombocytopenic; the following are offered as guidelines only:

1.   Open biopsies are generally safer than needle biopsies because
     of the ability to visually inspect for bleeding.

2.   In the absence of a concomitant clotting problem or a problem
     with platelet function, a platelet count greater than 50,000
     is usually associated with adequate platelet plug function.

3.   Even with higher platelet counts be wary if the patient
     demonstrates evidence of bleeding from venipunctures, etc.,
     or has a concomitant clotting problem (e.g., DIC or liver
     disease.

4.   With platelet counts less than 50,000 per ul bleeding from
     procedures is more likely to occur in patients with amegakaryo-
     cytic, production thrombocytopenias (leukemia, aplasia,
     myelophthisis) than thrombocytopenia due to increased platelet
     destruction or sequestration (e.g., ITP or hypersplenism).

5.   Lumbar puncture and needle organ biopsies (lung, liver,
     kidneys, etc.) are more hazardous than thoracentesis, paracen-
     tesis, bone marrow aspirate and biopsy. The "need to know"
     must be carefully assessed. In amegakaryocytic, production
     thrombocytopenia and platelet counts less than 50,000 per
     ul, platelet transfusions are indicated prior to and probably
     for several days following such procedures.

6.   Diagnostic needle procedures are hazardous in patients with
     platelet dysfunction no matter what the platelet count (see
     p. 81).

SUMMARY

Remember:

1. In severe thrombocytopenia (< 10,000) think of:

    a. Immune thrombocytopenia

    b. Aplastic anemia

    c. Acute leukemia

2. Large and frequently elongated platelets seen on a fingerstick
    smear are usually young platelets, and their presence suggests
    a destructive/sequestration mechanism for the thrombocytopenia.

3. The degree of bleeding at any given platelet count varies
    with mechanism.

    a. Production (amegakaryocytic) thrombocytopenia will
        frequently demonstrate significant bleeding with counts
        less than 20,000, whereas destructive/sequestration
        thrombocytopenias may not bleed at much lower counts.
        This feature is nicely demonstrated by the relationship
        of bleeding time (p. 82) and platelet count in the
        two mechanisms. The aplastic anemia patient with 10,000
        platelets will have markedly prolonged bleeding time,
        whereas the ITP patient with 10,000 platelets may have
        a normal bleeding time. The explanation for this vari-
        ability is thought to be related to the functional
        superiority of young platelets in comparison to old
        platelets. In any event the clinician is much more
        concerned about the likelihood of significant bleeding
        in severe production thrombocytopenia than in severe
        destruction/sequestration thrombocytopenia.

4. Platelet transfusions are used for severe production thrombo-
    cytopenia. They are not helpful, as a rule, in destruction/
    sequestration thrombocytopenia.

5. We have more platelets than we need. Hemostasis approaches
    normal at platelet counts greater than 50,000 in production
    thrombocytopenia and at lower counts in destruction/sequestration
    thrombocytopenia.

DISORDERS OF PLATELET FUNCTION

Hemostatic plug type clinical bleeding in the absence of thrombocytopenia raises the suspicion of the presence of an abnormality of
platelet function. The further data base for a suspected disorder

of platelet function frequently begins with a <u>bleeding time.</u>

The Bleeding Time

The <u>bleeding time</u> is a gross in vivo test of hemostatic plug function. Bleeding times based on the template method are accurate and disposable devices are commercially available (Hemakit, Simplate II). There is poor correlation between the degree of prolongation of the bleeding time and the degree of clinical bleeding, but the test is useful as a means to diagnose platelet dysfunction.

Normal Platelet Function

Following adherence of a few platelets to exposed collagen after vascular injury, normal hemostatic plug activity involves three major platelet functions.

1.   Release of platelet ADP resulting in secondary aggregation of platelets at the damaged vessel site.

2.   Generation of platelet thromboxane A_2, a potent aggregator of platelets and vasoconstrictor. Conversely, prostaglandin intermediates generated by platelets are metabolized in the vessel wall to prostacyclin (PGI_2), an antiaggregating agent and vasodilator (Fig.8.1).

3.   Platelet participation in clot formation. Several coagulation cascade reactions require platelet lipid and occur normally on the platelet membrane. These include reactions involving Factors XI, VIII, X and V. Platelets also contribute to clot formation by secreting stored clotting Factors I, V, VIII and XIII. Thrombin generated by the coagulation cascade is a potent platelet aggregator.

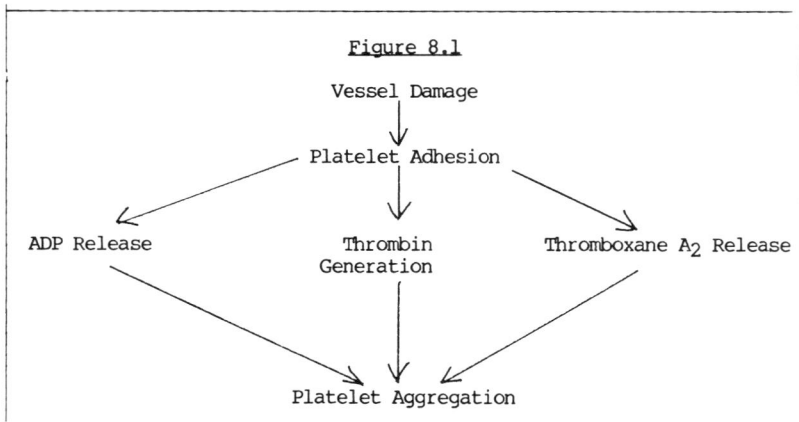

Figure 8.1

Vessel Damage

Platelet Adhesion

ADP Release   Thrombin Generation   Thromboxane A_2 Release

Platelet Aggregation

Disorders of Platelet Function

__Congenital__ causes of abnormal platelet function are quite rare (except for von Willebrand's disease). Several syndromes have been identified:

a. __von Willebrand's disease__ (p. 100).

b. __Bernard-Soulier syndrome__: An autosomal recessive disease characterized by large bizarre platelet morphology, mild thrombocytopenia and defective platelet adhesion secondary to an intrinsic membrane defect.

c. __Glanzmann's thrombasthenia__: Autosomal recessive disease associated with absent clot retraction and abnormal platelet aggregation.

d. __Disorders of ADP secretion__: A heterogeneous group of disorders characterized by defective aggregation secondary to abnormal ADP secretion.

__Acquired__ disorders of platelet function are much more common:

a. __Drugs__: ASA interferes with platelet function by inhibiting prostaglandin synthesis and the formation of thromboxane A_2. A prolonged bleeding time may be identified in normals following the ingestion of 1 or 2 aspirin tablets, and aspirin accentuates the bleeding time prolongation in patients with underlying disorders of platelet function. __Aspirin should not be given to patients with known bleeding disorders.__ Some of the penicillins may cause clinical bleeding associated with a markedly prolonged bleeding time especially in patients with renal failure or mild thrombocytopenia. Carbenicillin, penicillin, ampicillin, cephalothin and moxalactam all may significantly prolong the bleeding time and cause clinical bleeding. Alcohol may cause prolongation of the bleeding time. Although a large number of other agents have been shown to affect platelet function in vitro, few have actually been implicated as causing clinical bleeding.

Figure 8.2

Thromboxane A$_2$ Generation

Membrane Phospholipids

$\downarrow$

Arachidonic Acid

Cyclo Oxygenase

$\downarrow$

PGG$_2$
PGH$_2$

Platelet
Thromboxane A$_2$

Blood Vessel
Prostacyclin (PGI$_2$)

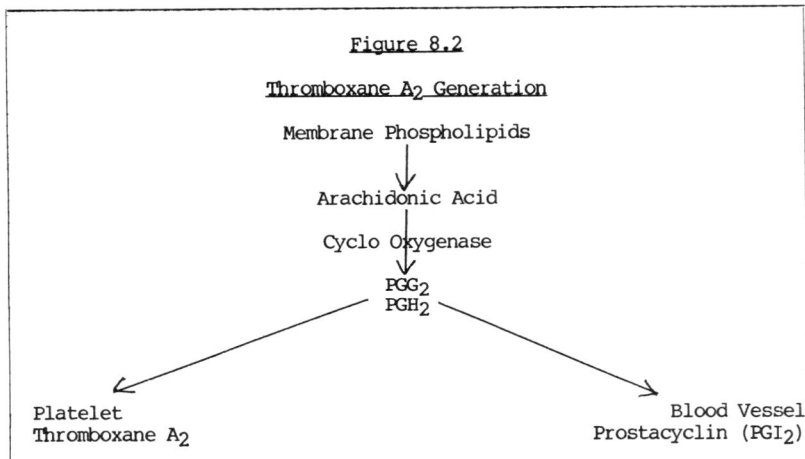

b. **Uremia:** Bleeding time prolongation associated with platelet dysfunction is seen in severe uremia (dialysis patients), probably due to metabolic byproducts. These may be removed by dialysis, which is the treatment of choice for severe hemostatic plug type bleeding in patients with renal failure. There are some reports suggesting that the transfusion of cryoprecipitate (perhaps as a source of von Willebrand factor, p. 100) may help to correct the platelet dysfunction prominent in some severely uremic patients. Infusion of 1-deamino-8-D-arginine vasopressin (DDAVP) which increases the plasma concentration of Factor VIII, von Willebrand Factor multimers (p. 101) has also been reported to temporarily correct the platelet dysfunction in uremia.

c. **Cardiopulmonary bypass surgery:** A marked bleeding time prolongation occurs during cardiopulmonary bypass secondary to oxygenator-induced platelet activation. When clinical bleeding occurs, platelet transfusion should be given.

d. **Miscellaneous:** Platelet dysfunction is seen in some patients with **severe liver disease** (perhaps related to high levels of fibrinogen/fibrin degradation products), patients with **multiple myeloma** and other **dysproteinemias** (proteins interfering with platelet function), and some patients with **leukemia** (abnormal platelet function). Patients with **chronic myeloproliferative disorders** and elevated platelet counts have functionally abnormal platelets as well.

THROMBOCYTOSIS

Table 8.7 lists the common etiologies of thrombocytosis. Chronic myeloproliferative disorders frequently are associated with platelet counts greater than 1,000,000 per μl. The platelets are morphologically bizarre and functionally abnormal. This is more common in polycythemia vera, primary myelofibrosis and primary thrombocythemia than in chronic granulocytic leukemia. Bleeding is common in such patients, usually when the platelet count is quite high. The platelets also tend to clump in the microcirculation and may contribute to the thrombotic problems seen in these patients. Many recommend treatment to decrease the platelet count in such patients (alkylating agents, ^{32}p), although proof of efficacy is difficult to determine. Secondary thrombocytosis does not cause a bleeding diathesis.

Table 8.7
Thrombocytosis: Differential Diagnosis

Myeloproliferative Disorders (frequently > 1,000,000)

    Polycythemia vera
    Primary thrombocythemia
    Agnogenic myeloid metaplasia
    Chronic granulocytic leukemia

Secondary Thrombocytosis

    Inflammation
    Malignancy
    Hodgkin's disease
    Acute bleeding
    Postsplenectomy
    Rebound from severe thrombocytopenia
    Severe iron deficiency

NONTHROMBOCYTOPENIC PURPURA WITH NORMAL PLATELET FUNCTION

Many of the following disorders are sometimes associated with skin and/or mucous membrane hemorrhage suggestive of a hemostatic plug type bleeding defect. However, others are associated with ecchymoses and confluent lesions more suggestive of a coagulation problem.

    Senile purpura
    Steroid purpura
    Connective tissue disorders (Ehlers-Danlos syndrome, pseudo-
      xanthoma elasticum)
    Scurvy

Amyloidosis
Dysproteinemias
Allergic purpura
Autoerythrocyte sensitization.

REFERENCES

Cohen I, Gardner FH: Thrombocytopenia as a laboratory sign and compli-
cation of gram negative bacteremia infection. Arch Intern Med
117:112, 1966.
Cowan DH, Henes JD: Thrombocytopenia of severe alcoholism. Ann Intern
Med 74:37, 1971.
Garg SK, Lackner H, Karpatkin S: The increased percentage of mega-
thrombocytes in various clinical disorders. Ann Intern Med
77:361, 1972.
Gynn TN, Mesmore HL, Friedman IA: Drug induced thrombocytopenia.
Med Clin North Am 56:65, 1972.
Harker LA, Finch CA: Thrombokinetics in man. J Clin Invest 48:963,
1969.
Harker LA, et al: Mechanism of abnormal bleeding in patients undergoing
cardiopulmonary bypass: acquired transient platelet dysfunction
associated with selective α-granule release. Blood 56:824-834,
1980.
Kelton, JG, Powers PJ, Carter CJ: A prospective study of the usefulness
of the measurement of platelet-associated IgG for the diagnosis
of ITP. Blood 60:1050-1053, 1982.
McMillan R: Chronic idiopathic thrombocytopenic purpura. N Engl
J Med 304:1135, 1981.
Molpass TW, Harker LA: Acquired disorders of platelet function.
Sem in Hematol 17:242-258, 1980.
Piscotta AV, et al: Treatment of thrombotic thrombocytopenic purpura
by exchange transfusion. Am J Hematol 3:71-82, 1977.

Chapter 9

Disorders of Clotting

Based on the results of the initial data base discussed in Chapter 5, the diagnostic focus narrows. This chapter deals with disorders of clotting, without evidence of an associated platelet problem.

<u>ISOLATED PROLONGATION OF THE aPTT</u>
<u>(NORMAL PT, TT AND PLATELET COUNT, FIG. 9.1)</u>

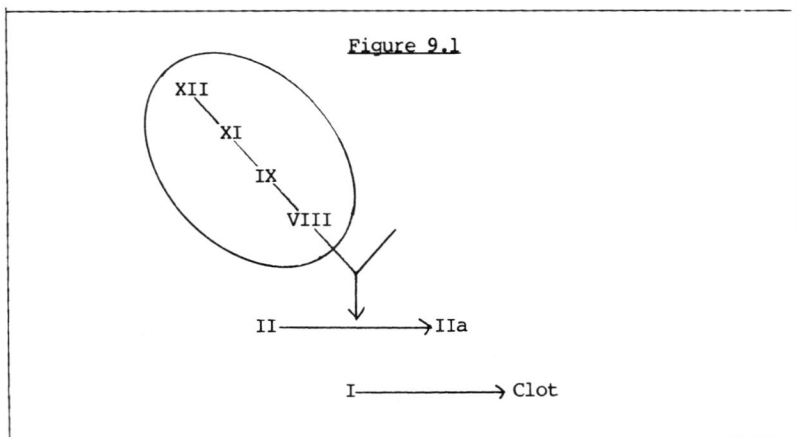

<u>Figure 9.1</u>

<u>Differential Diagnosis</u>

. Spurious

. Circulating anticoagulant

. von Willebrand's disease

87

- Hemophilia A and B

- Congenital deficiency of Factors XI and XII

- Congenital deficiency of Fletcher, Passovoy and Fitzgerald Factors

- Constant infusion heparin

Spurious

An unexpected prolongation of the aPTT is usually spurious and the test should be repeated with attention to proper filling of the tube (ratio of anticoagulant to blood is important and rapid transport to the lab for assay (p. 66). If the aPTT is still abnormal, it _must_ be explained even in the absence of a history of bleeding (see hemophilia below).

Circulating Anticoagulant

Differential Diagnosis

- Hemophilia A and B

- Postpartum

- Elderly

- SLE

- Drugs (chlorpromazine, penicillin)

Acquired inhibitors of coagulation factors may develop in the multiply transfused hemophiliac (anti-VIII/anti-IX), resulting usually in severe bleeding refractory to factor replacement. Inhibitors may develop spontaneously in women postpartum, rarely during the administration of various drugs (chlorpromazine, penicillin) and occasionally for no apparent reason in the elderly. These inhibitors are usually directed against Factor VIII, but occasionally against Factor IX, XI or V. An anti-VIII anticoagulant may develop in systemic lupus erythematosus, although usually the anticoagulant is directed against lipid and results in a slight prolongation of the PT as well as aPTT. Paradoxically patients with the lupus anticoagulant have a tendency to thrombosis rather than bleeding.

Treatment

If secondary to multiple transfusions in the hemophiliac, the circulating antibody may be quite serious and difficult to treat. Treatment attempts include:

1. Massive transfusion with appropriate factor concentrates

(VIII or IX).

2. Immunosuppression (of questionable effectiveness).

3. Induction of immunotolerance (European hemophilia centers).

4. In hemophilia A attempts to bypass the block by giving activated Factor X (FEIBA and Autoplex) have been effective.

In other settings, e.g., SLE, the anticoagulant may be of little consequence, although bleeding is sometimes seen. The anticoagulant is frequently transitory and rarely needs specific therapy.

von Willebrand's Disease (p. 100)

Von Willebrand's disease, discussed in Chapter 10, classically results in a prolonged bleeding time as well as in decreased Factor VIII activity (prolonged aPTT), but may yield only a prolonged aPTT in some patients. Diagnosis is usually suggested by a family history suggesting an autosomal dominant inheritance pattern and by a bleeding pattern more suggestive of a "hemostatic plug" formation problem in contrast to the hemophiliac.

Congenital Abnormalities of Coagulation

Approximately 85% of such patients have defective Factor VIII function, 12% have defective Factor IX function and 1% have Factor XI deficiency. (Deficiencies of Factor XII and Fletcher, Fitzgerald and Passovoy Factors are very rare.) Therefore, most patients (except for rare cases deficient in other coagulation factors) manifest a prolonged aPTT with a normal PT and TT. About 50% of cases are severe (< 2% activity for Factor VIII) and are diagnosed in infancy. However, mild cases (5-20% activity) are seen in persons who reach adult life without serious bleeding. Such patients may have life-threatening bleeding with trauma or surgery, hence, the obvious importance of explaining an unexpected prolongation of the aPTT. The aPTT is sensitive enough to detect procoagulant levels below 25% activity.

Concentrates of Factors VIII and IX may be used to treat major bleeds, but since they are prepared from large donor pools they carry a hepatitis risk. Recent reports of acquired immunodeficiency syndrome (AIDS) in hemophiliacs receiving concentrate (not cyroprecipitate) have added further concern. Cryoprecipitate units (p. 108) containing the concentrated Factor VIII from a single donor are safer and particularly useful for minor and moderate bleeds. Home transfusion programs, in which the patients administer cryoprecipitate or concentrate to themselves at the first evidence of a bleed (e.g., hemarthrosis) are particularly effective, as early transfusion prevents the late sequelae of delayed treatment of bleeding (e.g., joint destruction, contractions).

Constant Infusion Heparin (see p. 104)

Further Data Base

On the basis of the above comments, an unexpected prolongation of the aPTT might reasonably initiate the following workup:

a.   Repeat to rule out a spurious prolongation of the aPTT

b.   Screen for a circulating anticoagulant

c.   Assay of Factors VIII and IX

d.   Factor XI assay if the above are normal

e.   Testing to differentiate von Willebrand's disease from hemophilia (p. 100).

ISOLATED PROLONGATION OF THE PT OR PT AND aPTT
(NORMAL TT AND PLATELET COUNT, FIG. 9.2)

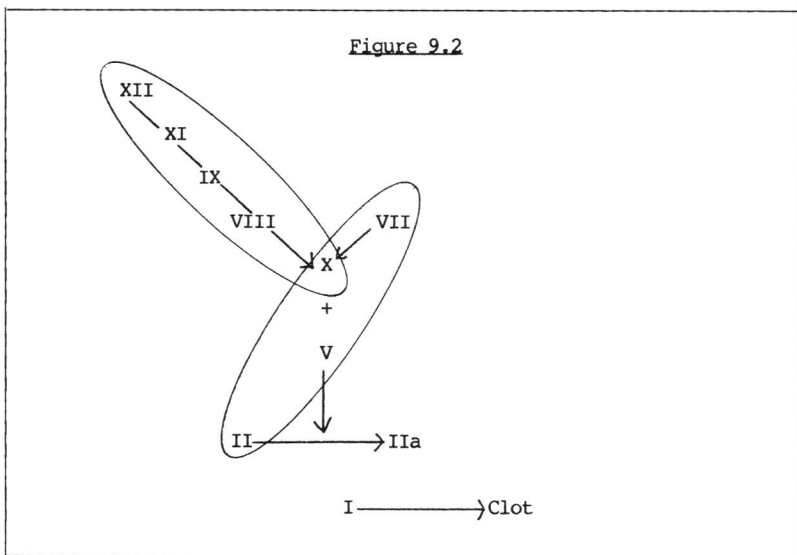

Figure 9.2

Differential Diagnosis

Coumarin anticoagulation

- Vitamin K deficiency

- Liver disease

- Rare congenital coagulation defects

- Circulating anticoagulant (SLE)

- Chronic DIC

- Excessive heparinization

- Aspirin

Coumadin Anticoagulation and Vitamin K Deficiency (see p. 105)

Liver Disease

Early hepatocellular disease may cause prolongation of the PT primarily due to decrease in Factor VII formation. With further worsening of liver function, the aPTT may become abnormal as well. Only in end-stage liver disease do fibrinogen levels fall significantly. In very severe hepatocellular disease the TT may be prolonged because of the liver's inability to clear fibrin split products, and a picture which suggests DIC may be seen (p. 94).

Congenital Coagulation Defects

Congenital deficiencies of Factor VII, Factor X, Factor V and Factor II occur rarely.

Circulating Anticoagulant

The common anticoagulant seen in SLE is directed against platelet lipid and prothrombin. Paradoxically patients with the "lupus anti-coagulant", may be more prone to thrombosis (perhaps because of inhibition of vessel wall prostacyclin synthesis), and in clinical settings associated with an increased thrombotic risk anticoagulation has been recommended.

DIC (p. 94)

Heparin (p. 103)

Aspirin

Salicylates in large doses may prolong the PT (and sometimes the PTT) probably because of an effect on prothrombin synthesis. Vitamin K prevents the abnormality. Bleeding is uncommon.

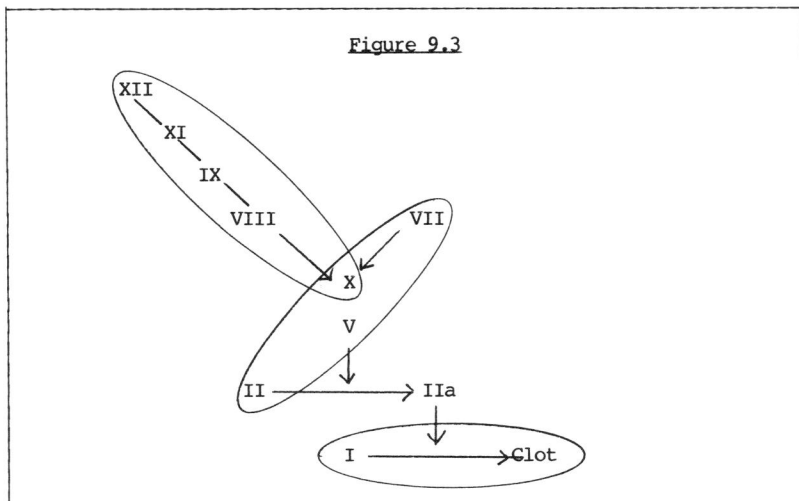

Figure 9.3

Third-stage coagulation problems characteristically prolong the thrombin time. The PT and aPTT are also abnormal because the endpoint of all three tests require a normal third stage for clot formation. Depending on the method, the thrombin time may be less sensitive than the PT and PTT and may be normal in some situations where there is abnormal third-stage coagulation.

Differential Diagnosis

. Afibrinogenemia (hypofibrinogenemia)

. Dysfibrinogenemia

. High dose heparin

. DIC

. Fibrinolysis

. Severe liver disease

. Paraproteinemia

Afibrinogenemia and Hypofibrinogenemia

These are rare hereditary disorders of blood coagulation. Severe hypofibrinogenemia may also be acquired secondary to fulminant acute intravascular clotting as in obstetric emergencies (retained dead fetus, amniotic fluid embolism).

Dysfibrinogenemia

Functionally abnormal fibrinogens occur as rare congenital disorders and may occasionally be seen as acquired problems in liver disease (especially hepatomas).

High Dose Heparin (p. 103)

DIC (p. 94)

Fibrinolysis (p. 107)

Severe Liver Disease

Paraproteinemia

Some patients with large concentrations of monoclonal proteins (myeloma, macroglobulinemia) develop coagulopathies secondary to inhibition by the protein of various steps in coagulation. Third-stage inhibition is most common, although any pattern, as well as platelet dysfunction, can be seen.

Hazards of Invasive Procedures

In general, invasive diagnostic or therapeutic procedures carry a significant risk of bleeding in patients with any of the above disorders of clotting. Abnormalities of the PT, PTT, or TT should be respected. A specific diagnosis should be pursued, appropriate consultation obtained and indicated therapy instituted prior to invasive procedures.

REFERENCES

Bennett B: Coagulation pathways: interrelationships and control mechanism. Semin Hematol 14:301, 1977.
Biggs R: Recent advances in the management of haemophilia and Christmas disease. Clin Haematol 8:95, 1979.
Lewis JH, Spero JA, Hasibi U: Coagulopathies. Dis Month June 1977.
Mueh JR, Herbst KD, Rapaport SI: Thrombosis in patients with the lupus anticoagulant. Ann Intern Med 92:156-159, 1980.
Roberts HR: Hemophiliacs with inhibitors. Therapeutic options. N Engl J Med 305:757-758, 1981.
Zieve, PD, Levin J: Disorders of Hemostasis. Philadelphia, WB Saunders, 1976.

Chapter 10

Conditions Associated with Abnormalities of both Clotting and Platelets

During the workup of a patient for a bleeding diathesis, the finding of evidence of abnormalities involving both clotting and platelets (quantitative or qualitative) suggests the presence of one of the following clinical problems:

Differential Diagnosis

.   DIC
.   Alcohol
.   Liver disease
.   von Willebrand's disease
.   Dilution coagulopathy

DISSEMINATED INTRAVASCULAR COAGULATION

Intravascular clotting may be initiated by release of thromboplastic substances into the circulation, activating clotting through the extrinsic system, as, for example, in malignancy or tissue ischemia secondary to hypotension.

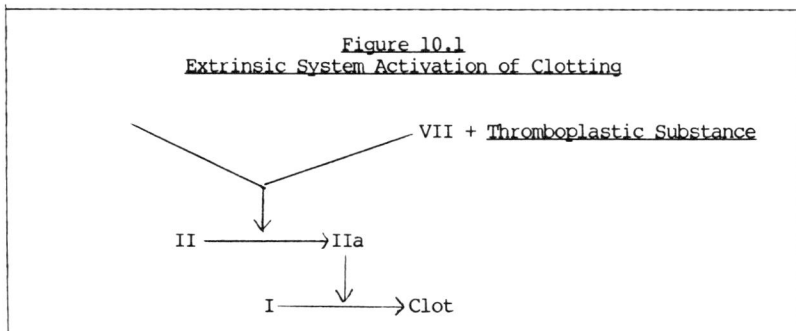

Figure 10.1
Extrinsic System Activation of Clotting

VII + Thromboplastic Substance

II ⟶ IIa

I ⟶ Clot

Clotting may also occur from activation of the intrinsic system, as for example from endotoxin in Gram-negative sepsis.

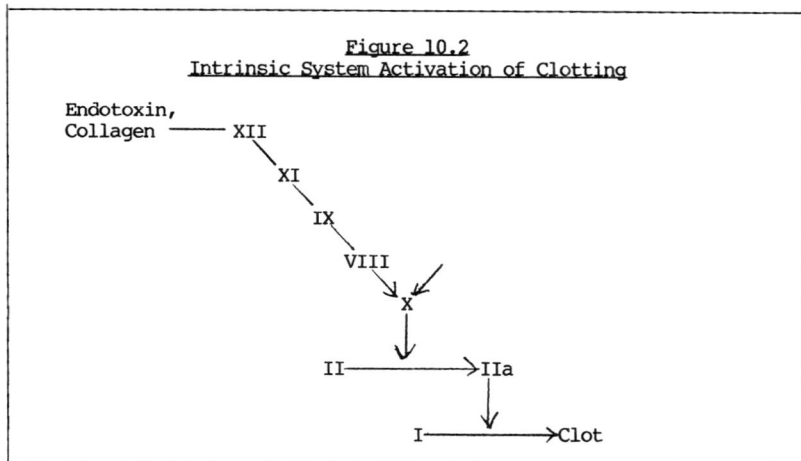

Figure 10.2
Intrinsic System Activation of Clotting

Endotoxin,
Collagen ——— XII
                    ＼
                     XI
                       ＼
                        IX
                          ＼
                           VIII   ↙
                               ↘↓ ↙
                                 X
                                 ↓
                   II————————→IIa
                                   ↓
                         I————————→Clot

Platelets are usually consumed in the clotting process. DIC may occur as an <u>acute</u> event or as a more <u>chronic</u> ongoing phenomenon.

Acute DIC

Table 10.1
Differential Diagnosis of Acute DIC

Obstetrics

    Retained dead fetus
    Amniotic fluid embolism
    Abrupto placentae
    Fatty liver of pregnancy
    Saline- or urea-induced abortion

Infection (bacterial, viral, rickettsial, mycotic, protozoal)
Shock
Acute progranulocytic leukemia
Hemolytic transfusion reactions
Heat stroke
Tissue necrosis
Leveen shunt

Acute DIC is usually severe, and there is frequently significant clinical bleeding.

<u>Laboratory Features</u>

a.   Various clotting factors are consumed (I, V, VIII, XIII)

b.   Platelets are consumed, and thrombocytopenia may be severe.

c.   Secondary fibrinolysis is activated.

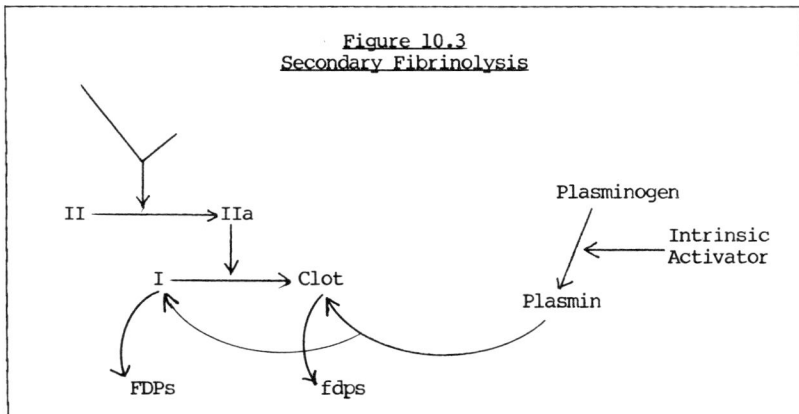

Figure 10.3
Secondary Fibrinolysis

Circulating plasminogen is activated to the enzyme plasmin, which digests fibrinogen and fibrin (as well as other coagulation factors, e.g., V and VIII), resulting in:

Fibrinogen degradation products (FDPs)
Fibrin degradation products (fdps)

FDPs/fdps circulate until cleared by the liver. They may be measured in vitro by one of several techniques. These products themselves interfere with normal clot formation (act as antithrombins and interfere with normal fibrin polymerization). They may also interfere with normal platelet function.

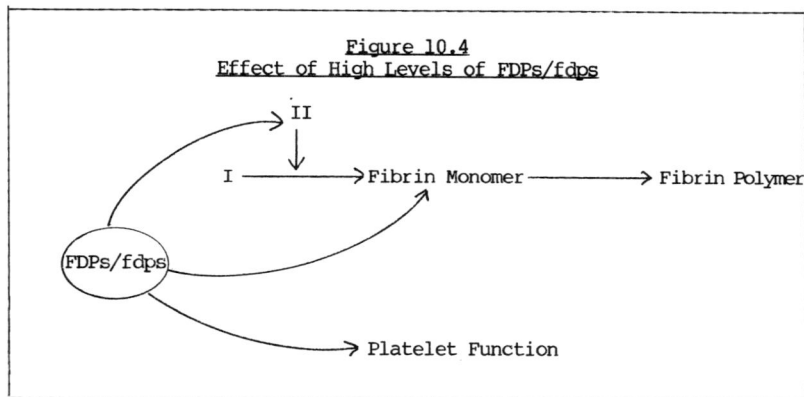

Figure 10.4
Effect of High Levels of FDPs/fdps

The bleeding in acute DIC results from a combination of problems:

1. Clotting factor consumption

2. Thrombocytopenia

3. Production of FDPs/fdps which act as anticoagulants.

Common Laboratory Data Base

1. PT - abnormal

2. aPTT - abnormal

3. TT - abnormal

4. Thrombocytopenia

5. Elevated levels of FDPs/fdps

6. Poor formation and/or lysis occurs when the clot is observed in vitro

7. RBC fragmentation (from fibrin deposition in arterioles) occurs in a minority of cases

Once the process of intravascular clotting is stopped (usually by eliminating the underlying cause), there is a rapid reversal of the abnormal laboratory tests. The PTT, aPTT and TT may return toward normal in a matter of hours, and FDPs/fdps are rapidly cleared by the liver. The platelet count returns to normal more slowly (over several days).

Subacute DIC

A less fulminant degree of intravascular clotting may occur in all of the causes of DIC listed above. In such cases the degree of abnormality seen in the laboratory data is quite variable, and the diagnosis becomes more difficult. Most hematologists require at least the following laboratory abnormalities for diagnosis:

1.   Decrease in the fibrinogen concentration

2.   At least a mild thrombocytopenia

3.   Elevated FDPs/fdps

Chronic DIC

The best clinical example of chronic DIC is metastatic cancer. Low levels of ongoing intravascular clotting probably explain other hypercoagulable phenomena seen frequently in cancer patients, namely, migrating thrombophlebitis and marantic endocarditis. The process of DIC in such patients may be mild and compensated, and clinical bleeding is infrequent. Diagnosis may be difficult.

Routine Laboratory Tests

1.   PT – normal or slightly abnormal

2.   aPTT – normal or slightly abnormal

3.   TT – normal or slightly abnormal

4.   Platelet count – frequently normal or even elevated

5.   FDPs/fdps – elevated

6.   Clot appearance in vitro – frequently normal

Remember that less fulminant DIC may be hard to diagnose and may result in only minor routine laboratory abnormalities. Extremely low-grade DIC may only be detected by sensitive tests of fibrinogen and platelet survival. Less fulminant DIC may be extremely difficult to distinguish from liver disease or from the dilution coagulopathy seen in the massively transfused patient.

Treatment

By far the most important treatment is that directed at the cause. Treat the shock, sepsis, or evacuate the dead fetus, etc. Intravascular coagulation may be interrupted by heparin administration (acts as an antithrombin and inhibits Factor X activation). Once clot formation is stopped, fibrinolysis ceases and FDPs/fdps are no longer formed.

Replacement therapy in patients with severe thrombocytopenia/hypofibrin-ogenemia is usually recommended if there is significant bleeding or surgery is needed. Platelets and fresh frozen plasma (or cryoprecipitate if the hypofibrinogenemia is severe) are given. Heparin is usually

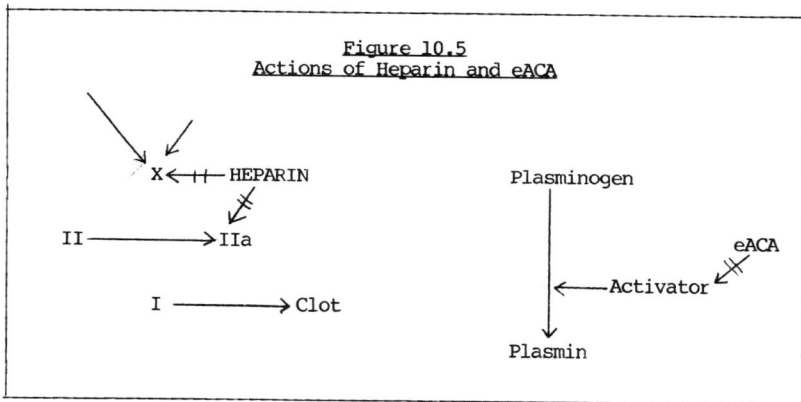

Figure 10.5
Actions of Heparin and eACA

recommended in patients with thrombotic complications of DIC (e.g., digital ischemia in purpura fulminans, thromboembolism) and in patients with progranulocytic leukemia undergoing treatment. Its use in other causes of DIC is controversial. There are no good controlled studies showing efficacy of treatment with heparin. As noted, the diagnosis in subacute cases may have considerable side effects. Acute cases are frequently rapidly reversible by treatment of the underlying cause.

LIVER DISEASE AND ALCOHOL

It is common for one to see abnormalities of both clotting and platelets in the setting of acute liver disease and/or alcoholism. Bleeding may occur for multiple reasons:

1. Decreased production of factors made in the liver (II, VII, V, IX, X).

2. Decreased production of vitamin K factors in obstructive jaundice (II, VII, IX, X).

3. Low-grade DIC with decreased clearance of FDPs/fdps.

4. Thrombocytopenia from:

   Hypersplenism

DIC

ETOH alone

Folate deficiency, especially in the alcoholic.

von Willebrand's Disease

This is an autosomal dominant disease with marked variability in degree of clinical bleeding. The bleeding pattern is more like that of a hemostatic plug defect than a clotting problem, with gastrointestinal bleeding being most common. Hemarthroses are usually not seen.

Pathophysiology

Functional Factor VIII results from the interaction of two molecular complexes, one x-linked defective in Hemophilia A and one under autosomal control (Factor VIII/von Willebrand Factor, F VIII/vWF) which is abnormal in von Willebrand's disease. F VIII/vWF is produced by the endothelial lining cells of blood vessels and is necessary for normal platelet/endothelial cell interaction. Von Willebrand's disease is not a single entity. Quantitative (Type I) and Qualitative (Type II A and B) abnormalities in F VIII/vWF have been described.

Routine Laboratory Findings

- Prolonged bleeding time. Accentuated by aspirin.

- Frequently (not always) prolonged aPTT.

- Normal PT, TT, platelet count.

Specialized Laboratory Tests

- Plasma Factor VIII procoagulant (VIII:co) activity (decreased in Type I disease; normal or decreased in Types II A and II B).

- Plasma Factor VIII-related antigen (VIII R:Ag) activity (decreased in Type I; normal or decreased in Types IIA and IIB).

- Plasma Factor VIII-related ristocetin cofactor (VIII R:R co) activity (decreased in Types I and II A and usually decreased in Type II B).

- Electrophoresis of F VIII/vWF by various techniques.

Treatment

Fresh frozen plasma (FFP) and cryoprecipitate are frequently effective in correcting the aPTT and bleeding time abnormalities and the clinical bleeding. Lyophilized Factor VIII concentrates do not correct the platelet function abnormality. Because of the large quantity of FFP required, cryoprecipitate has evolved as the treatment of choice. The amount necessary varies from patient to patient. Commonly 6 to 12 units given daily or every other day are required. Infusion of 1–deamino–8–D–arginine vasopressin (DDAVP) increases the plasma concentration of F VIII/vWF and may temporarily correct the bleeding diathesis in some patients (especially Type I) with von Willebrand's disease.

DILUTION COAGULOPATHY

This problem is seen particularly in trauma patients undergoing massive transfusions with banked blood. Blood refrigerated in the blood bank for 10 days to 3 weeks becomes depleted of:

- Functioning platelets (depleted in 1 day)

- Factor VIII

- Factor V

Dilution in vivo of platelets and Factors V and VIII may result in:

- Thrombocytopenia

- Prolongation of PT

- Prolongation of aPTT

- Associated clinical bleeding

Treatment

Treatment consists of appropriate, preferably preventive, replacement of platelets, Factor V and Factor VIII. In an adult it is reasonable to substitute a unit of fresh whole blood for every 4 units of old banked blood after the use of 10 units of old banked blood in a 24-hour period. It is difficult for the blood bank to supply fresh blood, and, therefore, one may substitute a unit of platelets, a unit of FFP (containing Factors VIII and V) and a unit of packed cells for a unit of fresh whole blood.

Comments

In the controlled setting of hypertransfusion (e.g., open heart surgery) it is unusual to see marked thrombocytopenia, a significant prolongation of the PT and PTT and clinical bleeding even with massive transfusion. In the trauma patient frequently in shock one sees more abnormal numbers and a more marked bleeding diathesis, usually because DIC is also present and diagnostically difficult to distinguish from dilution coagulopathy.

Table 10.2
Laboratory Comparison of Various States Causing Abnormalities
in both Clotting and Platelets

	PT	PTT	TT	Platelets	FDPs/fdps
Acute DIC	Abnl.	Abnl.	Abnl.	Decreased	Increased
Chronic DIC	May be normal	May be normal	May be normal	May be normal	Increased
Severe Liver Disease	Abnl.	Abnl.	May be abnl.	May be decreased (hyper-splenism)	Frequently increased
von Willebrand's Disease	Normal	Frequently abnl.	Normal	Normal (abnl. function)	Normal
Dilution Coagulopathy	Abnl.	Abnl.	Normal	Decreased	Normal

REFERENCES

Counts RB, et al: Hemostasis in massively transfused trauma patients. Ann Surg 190:91–99, 1979.

Feinstein D: Diagnosis and management of disseminated intravascular coagulation: the role of heparin therapy. Blood 60:284–287, 1982.

Ruggeri ZM, et al: Multimeric composition of Factor VIII/von Willebrand Factor following administration of DDAVP: Implications for pathophysiology and therapy of von Willebrand's disease subtypes. Blood 59:1272–1278, 1982.

Chapter 11

Anticoagulation

Method

Heparin has a short intravenous half-life (60-90 minutes), resulting in marked variability in the degree of coagulation when this drug is given by an intermittent injection regimen (intravenous or subcutaneous). Most experts consider the method of choice to be continuous intravenous infusion, preferably utilizing a constant flow rate infusion pump.

A loading dose of heparin is given (5,000-10,000 units) followed by a constant intravenous infusion (around 1,000 units per hour).

Monitoring

There is no ideal method for monitoring heparin dose. The clotting time used for several decades is subject to innumerable variables which are difficult to control. It is still used by many. There are various recommendations about the desired anticoagulant range (e.g. 2-3 ½ times, but a minimum of 20 minutes and a maximum of 40 minutes).

The aPTT has acquired many advocates in the last few years. However, various commercial aPTT systems use different thromboplastin substances. This results in considerable variability in the relationship between aPTT and the heparin dose. Some aPTT systems are not suitable for monitoring heparin dose. Some studies have shown no disadvantage in terms of recurrent thrombosis and bleeding complications when heparinization is not monitored at all. Most physicians, however, monitor heparin by either the CT or the aPTT.

An occasional patient is very resistant to heparin, especially during the first few days after a thrombotic event. Monitoring at this time is important in order to recognize the need for an increased heparin dose.

Monitoring recommendations:

1. For constant infusion heparinization use the aPTT if there has been in your hospital an assessment of the relationship (in vitro and in vivo) between the aPTT system used and the heparin concentration/dose.

2. If the above assessment has not been conducted use the clotting time, attempting to keep the range between 20 and 40 minutes.

3. With intermittent intravenous heparinization use the clotting time obtained just before the next heparin infusion (20-40 minutes).

Complications

Bleeding complications occur in 8-25% of heparinized patients. Minor bleeding problems predominate, but severe bleeds do occur (perhaps 1-2% of patients) and may include retroperitoneal, gastrointestinal and central nervous system bleeding. There is some suggestion that bleeding is less common in patients receiving continuous infusion rather than intermittent heparin.

Thrombocytopenia has been noted as a relatively common complication of heparin in several reports. For most of the cases the mechanism appears to be destructive possibly antibody mediated. When it occurs, thrombocytopenia usually begins shortly after heparinization. It may be severe, requiring discontinuation of treatment. Arterial thromboses sometimes accompany the syndrome of heparin thrombocytopenia. There is in vitro evidence that heparin potentiates platelet aggregation, raising another possible mechanism for thrombocytopenia in patients on heparin.

Because of heparin's half-life, the primary treatment for heparin-induced bleeding is transfusion support as needed and time, as the effects of anticoagulation will be gone in a few hours. Protamine may be given at a dose of 50 mg slowly intravenously. However, protamine in excess acts as an anticoagulant itself, and the exact dose needed to neutralize the circulating heparin is difficult to determine.

Low-dose Heparin

A number of clinical studies have suggested the efficacy of giving heparin in low doses intermittently as a useful way to prevent venous clotting in high-risk patients. Many physicians routinely treat post-myocardial infarction patients, patients after major surgery, and other bedridden or sedentary groups of patients with low-dose heparin. Doses recommended have been in the range of 5,000 units every 12 hours given subcutaneously. Bleeding problems are rare but may occur; monitoring is not necessary. This regimen is not effective in the treatment of established thromboembolic disease.

COUMARIN ANTICOAGULATION

Method

Coumarin anticoagulants inhibit the formation of Factors II, VII, IX and X by the liver. Warfarin (Coumadin) is the most commonly used coumarin anticoagulant and is given orally as one daily dose. The time necessary to reach appropriate anticoagulation is usually several days because of the long half-lives of several of the factors. Factor X (half-life of 24 hours) is decreased to the lowest level of all the factors in patients on chronic warfarin therapy. Factor VII, because of its short half-life (4 hours), is depressed rapidly, prolonging the prothrombin time within a day or two, especially when a large initial dose (loading dose) of warfarin is given. This phenomenon creates a false sense of security, since it is the level of Factor X in its pivotal position in both the intrinsic and extrinsic systems (p. 67) which is believed to be the most important guide to appropriate anticoagulation. Presently it is recommended, in the adult, that warfarin be given in a regular daily dose of 10-15 mg per day with the achievement of adequate anticoagulation occurring, on an average, 5 days from the initiation of treatment.

Dose Variability

Some patients are extremely resistant to Coumadin and may require as high as 20 mg or more daily. Others are extremely sensitive and may require only 2.5 mg two or three times a week.

A number of other factors beside host variability may affect warfarin dosage. The following factors enhance the effect of the drug:

1. Decreased vitamin K intake. Be careful in patients not eating for several days (e.g., postoperative patients), especially if they are on antibiotics which will decrease bacterial vitamin K production in the intestine.

2. Drugs which decrease albumin binding of drug. Those proven to affect anticoagulation in humans are chloral hydrate, phenylbutazone and oxyphenbutazone.

3. Liver disease decreases warfarin metabolism as well as causing decreased synthesis of vitamin K-dependent clotting factors. Note that severe congestive heart failure may affect this liver function also.

4. Drugs which potentiate warfarin effect by other than displacement from albumin include quinidine and anabolic steroids.

5. Discontinuation of those drugs which enhance warfarin metabolism: barbiturates, glutethimide, griseofulvin.

Monitoring

The one-stage prothrombin time is used to measure the effect of warfarin. It is sensitive to Factors II, VII and X. Factor IX levels, affected by warfarin, are not measured by the prothrombin time. The desired anticoagulation range is usually considered to be $1\frac{1}{2}$ -2 $\frac{1}{2}$ times the prothrombin time control range in seconds, but it varies with the individual method ($1\frac{1}{2}$-2 times control being appropriate with some methods).

Bleeding Complications

Bleeding is more likely when the patient is overanticoagulated but may occur when the prothrombin time is in the appropriate range. One should search for structural causes when GI and urinary bleeding occur. It is recommended that aspirin be avoided in patients on warfarin or heparin.

Once bleeding occurs, it may take 12-24 hours for vitamin K to correct the bleeding diathesis. Plasma contains the missing factors and should be given (3-4 units in an adult) when rapid correction of the bleeding diathesis is needed. Fresh frozen plasma is usually used, as this is usually the blood bank's only available source of single unit plasma. However, the prothrombin complex factors are maintained in aged nonfrozen plasma. Vitamin K should be given intravenously (to avoid intramuscular bleeding) and must be given at a slow rate of infusion to avoid hypotension (no faster than 3-5 mg per minute); 25-30 mg should be given (sometimes even larger doses are necessary).

Other Complications

1. Soon after initiation of treatment, rare patients may develop hemorrhagic infarcts, usually of the skin, with subsequent necrosis.

2. "Purple toes" syndrome. Less serious discoloration of the feet, seen mainly in men, which is transitory and not due to bleeding.

SWITCHING FROM HEPARIN TO COUMADIN

It takes approximately 5 days on an average to anticoagulate a patient with warfarin. Heparin is continued during this period. Patients receiving heparin by continuous infusion are more easily monitored during this period, as the prothrombin time is usually not prolonged by the blood heparin concentrations achieved with this method of heparinization. Therefore, the prothrombin time adequately reflects the state of warfarin anticoagulation. When heparin is given by an intermittent intravenous regimen, the prothrombin time is prolonged (sometimes for several hours) after heparin administration. In this situation it is best to omit a heparin dose and check the prothrombin time just before the next heparin injection.

	CT	PT	aPTT
Low-dose heparin	Normal	Normal	May be prolonged
Intermittent IV heparin			
at 30 min	Infinity	Markedly prolonged	Markedly prolonged
at 4 hours	20–40 min	Normal or slightly prolonged	1½–2½ times normal
Constant infusion heparin	20–40 min	Normal	1½–2½ times normal

Table 11.1
Effect of Appropriate Anticoagulation on Common
Tests of Coagulation

Thrombolytic Therapy

Preparations

Streptokinase and urokinase, activators of the fibrinolytic system have undergone extensive clinical testing and may be useful in the treatment of in vivo thrombosis. Streptokinase is available as a lyophilized concentrate containing 250,000 IU to 750,000 IU per vial. Urokinase is available as a lyophilized concentrate containing 250,000 IU per vial. Urokinase is usually reserved for use in patients who have antistreptokinase antibodies preventing a fibrinolytic effect from streptokinase (from prior streptococcal infections or prior treatment with streptokinase).

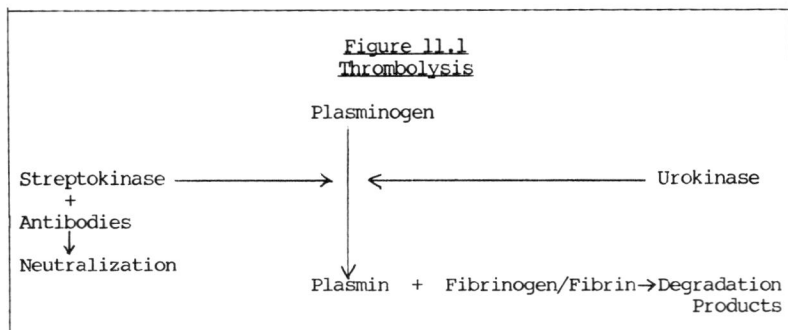

Figure 11.1
Thrombolysis

Plasminogen

Streptokinase ————————→   ←———————————— Urokinase
  +
Antibodies
  ↓
Neutralization   ↓
                       Plasmin + Fibrinogen/Fibrin→Degradation
                                                     Products

Rationale

Systemic fibrinolytic therapy rapidly dissolves recent in vivo clots (present less than 7 days) and, when compared to heparin therapy, more rapidly reverses thrombosis induced pulmonary and lower extremity vascular hypertension. It is reasonable to think that these efforts are beneficial in patients with pulmonary emboli (especially those with severe hemodynamic sequelae), although an effect on survival has not been proven. There is evidence that fibrinolytic therapy better preserves valves in the deep venous system in patients with proximal phlebitis when compared with heparin therapy; also, it may decrease the incidence of the post-phlebitic syndrome in patients with extensive deep vein thrombosis, although this is not well proven. Antifibrinolytic therapy may also be useful in the treatment of acute arterial thrombosis and acute thrombosis of arteriovenous shunts. Appropriate use of fibrinolytic therapy is still in the process of being defined.

Method for inducing systemic fibrinolysis with streptokinase.

A loading dose of 250,000 IU of streptokinase is given over 20-30 minutes through a peripheral line using a constant infusion pump. Febrile reactions with streptokinase occur frequently, and some recommend pretreatment with steroids (e.g., hydrocortisone 100 mg q 12 h during the fibrinolytic therapy). Streptokinase, 100,000 units per hour, is given by infusion pump for 24 hours for pulmonary embolism (PE) and for 48-72 hours for proximal deep vein thrombosis (DVT).

Table 11.2
Stepwise Procedure for Thrombolytic Therapy

1. Documented PE, DVT, etc., less than 7 days old.
2. Baseline thrombin time.
3. If heparinized, discontinue and wait until thrombin time is less than 2 times control.
4. Streptokinase 250,000 IU by infusion pump over 20-30 minutes (urokinase 4000 IU/kg over 30 minutes).
5. Streptokinase 100,000 IU/hr by infusion pump (urokinase 4000 units/kg/hour).
[a]6. Thrombin time at 4 hours, two to five times control.

   a. If less than 2 times control, discontinue fibrinolytic therapy and heparinize.
   b. If greater than 7 times control, discontinue therapy and check hourly. When less than five times control, start therapy back at half dose.

7. Following Rx (24 hours for PE, 48-72 hours for DVT), start constant infusion heparin when aPTT is two times control.

[a]Complicated and debated. See Koch-Weser, 1982.

Monitoring

The necessity of close monitoring is not proven. However, monitoring is necessary to prove fibrinolytic effect. A number of monitoring tests may be used (thrombin time, prothrombin time, partial thromboplastin time, euglobin lysis time, assay of fibrin degradation products). The objective is some prolongation compared to the pretreatment control. Some recommend maintaining the thrombin time (the most widely used monitor) between two and five times the control value. Constant infusion heparin should be instituted post fibrinolytic therapy when the aPTT is appropriately prolonged. Heparin is continued for the usual treatment period.

Contraindications and complications

Table 11.3 lists contraindications to thrombolytic therapy. Prolonged pressure should be applied when minor bleeding is experienced at previous venous and arterial puncture sites. More severe bleeding requires discontinuation of thrombolytic therapy and transfusion of plasma or cryoprecipitate. E-Aminocaproic acid is added for serious hemorrhage.

Table 11.3
Contraindications to Fibrinolytic Therapy

Absolute Contraindications

Acute internal hemorrhage
Recent intracranial process

Relative Contraindications

Major surgery, organ biopsy, delivery within 20 days
Recent serious trauma
Recent GI hemorrhage
Severe hypertension
Hemorrhagic retinopathy
Pregnancy
Hemorrhagic diathesis
Bacterial endocarditis
Presence of probable left heart thrombus

REFERENCES

Bell WR, Royall RM: Heparin-associated thrombocytopenia: a comparison
    of three heparin preparations. N Engl J Med 303:902-907, 1980.
Brozoric M: Oral anticoagulants in clinical practice. Semin Hematol
    15:27, 1978.
Deykin D: The use of heparin. N Engl J Med 280:937, 1969.
Deykin D: Warfarin therapy. N Engl J Med 283:691, 801, 1970.
Deykin D: Current status of anticoagulant therapy. Amer J Med 72:659-
    664, 1982.
Koch-Weser J: Thrombolytic therapy. N Engl J Med 304:1268-1276,
    1982.

Chapter 12

Blood Transfusion

TREATMENT OF ANEMIA

Remember the following when considering the need for red cell transfusion:

1. When anemia develops gradually, a number of compensating processes occur which diminish symptoms: shift of O_2 dissociation curve, various cardiovascular adjustments and an increase in plasma volume (and total blood volume). The elderly patient with a treatable, slowly developing chronic anemia (e.g., pernicious anemia, iron deficiency) who is asymptomatic at rest is best treated without transfusion. Volume overload (pulmonary edema) from transfusion is common in this situation.

2. Indications for transfusion in the above setting include:

    a. Angina pectoris

    b. Ischemic EKG changes

    c. High output congestive heart failure

    d. Organic cerebral symptoms

    e. Inability to keep the patient sedentary

3. Rapid bleeding may result in significant loss of blood volume without a drop in hematocrit. Beware of the patient with gastrointestinal bleeding and a normal hematocrit. Transfuse early.

RED CELL COMPONENTS

Whole Blood

This component is used infrequently. It is primarily indicated

111

for the actively bleeding patient with evidence of a decreased blood volume. Less acute bleeding (e.g., blood loss from surgery or mild gastrointestinal bleeding) can be managed by transfusion of packed cells.

Packed Red Blood Cells

Prepared from freshly drawn blood allowing preparation of plasma components (e.g., cryoprecipitate) and platelet units. Remember that the hematocrit of this product (depending on method of preparation) is around 70%, not 95%. There is appreciable plasma (albumin) left in this component. Packed cells given rapidly to the patient with a chronic anemia can precipitate pulmonary edema.

White Cell-poor Blood Components

Prepared in various ways (separation of buffy coat, washing, frozen red cells), these components are indicated primarily to avoid chills and fever from leukoagglutinin reactions in multiply transfused patients. The preparation of these units presents problems to the blood bank in terms of increased preparation time and the fact that they must be prepared from fresh or frozen blood. In addition, if washing is the method used to remove the white cells, the unit must be transfused within 24 hours of the washing procedure.

Fresh Blood

This usually refers to blood less than 6 hours old. When blood is stored in the refrigerator (currently, blood has a 21-day storage life before it must be transfused or discarded), a storage injury occurs resulting in loss of functional platelets (24 hours), loss of coagulation Factors V (1 week) and VIII (48 hours), a rise in plasma potassium from cell lysis, a decrease in red cell ATP and 2,3-DPG (resulting in an unfavorable shift of the O_2 dissociation curve) and, with time, significant loss of red cells (up to 30% at 3 weeks). With the use of newer anticoagulants and additives, many of these storage injuries are minimized except for the loss of coagulation factors and platelets. Appropriate uses of fresh blood include:

1. Massively transfused patients (10 or more units of old banked blood transfused within a 24-hour period in an adult). It is reasonable to supply 1 unit of fresh blood for every 4 units of old blood after the first 10 units transfused in order to prevent dilution of coagulation factors and platelets. Note the logistic difficulty for the blood bank to supply fresh whole blood. A unit of fresh frozen plasma, a platelet unit and a unit of packed red cells may be substituted for 1 unit of fresh blood.

2. Many pediatricians feel fresh blood is indicated in the

transfusion of the newborn to avoid hyperkalemia.

Frozen Red Cells

Frozen blood allows for a long storage life. It is useful for storing rare blood types and collecting blood for autotransfusion in the patient scheduled for elective surgery or the patient who may require the transfusion of rare blood types. It is an excellent source of white cell-poor blood.

PLATELET COMPONENTS

As discussed in Chapter 8, the treatment of thrombocytopenia differs with the mechanism. Platelet transfusions are reserved, in general, for severe production thrombocytopenia and are mainly used in the support of patients undergoing intensive chemotherapy. Available components include:

Random Single-donor Platelets

This component consists of platelets harvested from a single unit of fresh blood by centrifugation techniques and concentrated in 30-50 cc of donor plasma. This product has a short storage life (less than 3 days) and preferably should be used the day prepared. In an adult 1 unit of single-donor platelets will raise the platelet count around 6,000-12,000 per ul measured 1 hour post-transfusion. Increments are decreased in the setting of infection, fever, bleeding or sensitization from past transfusions.

HLA Identical Platelets

HLA identical platelets are indicated in the multiply transfused patient who has become sensitized to platelet antigens (primarily HLA antigens) and who no longer achieves a significant rise in platelet count with transfusion of random platelets. Such platelets are frequently given to prevent sensitization in the patient who will require future transfusion support. HLA identical platelets are usually obtained from a sibling by plateletphoresis. Platelet numbers comparable to 6-10 units of single-donor platelets may be harvested in 2-3 hours from a donor using special centrifugation techniques. Patients may be supported through severe aplasia by platelets harvested from a single donor, donating three times a week.

Frozen Platelets

Technology for freezing platelets is still imperfect and has lagged far behind red cell technology. A frozen platelet capability is greatly needed in order to facilitate longer storage life and improve the logistics of obtaining adequate numbers of platelets for transfusion.

OTHER COMPONENTS

Fresh Frozen Plasma (FFP)

Plasma is separated from fresh blood and stored at temperatures of -20°C or less. This product maintains activity of labile coagulation Factors V and VIII. Routine single-donor plasma contains other coagulation factors (including prothrombin complex Factors II, VII, IX and X). It is stored at 4°C and is stable in storage for long periods. However, the blood bank usually only stores single-donor plasma as FFP. Note that heat-treated plasma products such as "plasma protein fraction" do not contain coagulation factors. Appropriate indications for FFP include:

1. Prevention of dilution coagulopathy in the massively transfused patient.

2. Rapid correction of the coagulation abnormalities in the patient on warfarin.

3. Treatment of various congenital coagulation factor deficiencies (Factors IX, XI, VII, X, V deficiency).

4. Treatment of von Willebrand's disease.

Cryoprecipitate

Plasma separated from fresh blood is rapidly frozen at -90°C and then allowed to warm slowly at 4°C. Once rewarmed, most of the plasma is removed. A gelatinous precipitate is left suspended in a few milliliters of plasma, and the unit is stored at -20°C or less. This precipitate contains most of the Factor VIII and fibrinogen of the original plasma unit. Appropriate indications for cryoprecipitate include:

1. Treatment of hemophilia A (Factor VIII deficiency).

2. Treatment of von Willebrand's disease.

3. Treatment of hypofibrinogenemia.

White Cells for Transfusion

Special leukophoresis techniques are used to harvest white cells from donors by continuous or intermittent centrifugation. Donors are usually HLA identical family members supplying cells for patients with chemotherapy-induced bone marrow aplasia.

COMMON TRANSFUSION PROBLEMS ENCOUNTERED BY THE HOUSE OFFICER

An Urgent Need for Blood for a Patient Who Is Exsanguinating

When there is not enough time to complete a cross match, the blood bank will supply type-specific (ABO and Rh) blood. Remember that this requires a properly labeled cross match tube. It will take less than 5 minutes to determine the ABO and Rh type of the patient. The house officer will have to sign a release stating the blood is needed as an emergency before a cross match can be completed (the latter takes 45 minutes to 1 hour to complete).

Uncommon Blood Type, Urgent Need

The blood bank may not have enough AB-negative, AB-positive, B-negative blood, etc., to fulfill the needs of an exsanguinating trauma patient. Here one may have to use blood that is not the patient's type. The following is a guide:

1. AB-negative patient:

   O-negative blood is preferable. AB-positive or O-positive blood may be used if there is time to complete a cross-match to rule out the possibility of prior Rh sensitivity from a necessary previous transfusion of Rh-positive blood. Remember that, once the Rh-positive blood has been transfused to a Rh-negative recipient, sensitization is likely (less so in severely ill cancer patients on chemotherapy), and future transfusion with Rh-positive blood must be avoided.

2. AB-positive patient:

   Any type may be used. O-positive and A-positive are likely to be the easiest to obtain.

3. B-negative patient:

   O-negative blood is preferable. B-positive and O-positive may be used with the cautions mentioned above.

Notification by the Blood Bank That the Cross Match Tube Was Unlabeled

The most common cause of a severe hemolytic transfusion reaction, which carries high mortality, is misidentification resulting in the wrong blood being given to a patient. Blood bank rules about labeling of cross match tubes are not and should not be negotiable. As a corollary, when the physician hangs blood, he or she should follow the blood bank's guidelines for patient and blood identification to the letter and should have a nurse to repeat the check.

Notification by the Blood Bank That the Patient Has a Positive Direct Coombs' Test

See Chapter 4, p. 35.

Notification by the Blood Bank That the Patient Has a Positive Antibody Screen with Cross Matching Difficulties

See Chapter 4, p. 35.

COMMON TRANSFUSION REACTIONS

Table 12.1 Transfusion Reactions		
	Hemolytic	Leukoagglutinin
Incidence	Rare (1 in 5000 transfusions)	Common (3% of all transfusions)
Classic clinical	Arm pain, chest pain, back pain, shock, dia-phoresis; may be only chills and fever	Chills and fever
Time of symptoms	Early in transfusion	Late in transfusion
Plasma/urine	Red (brown); free hemoglobin	Normal
Fatality	High fatality	Almost never fatal

Hemolytic Reactions

Immediate hemolytic transfusion reactions are quite rare and are usually due to errors in patient or blood identification (or both). Classical features include:

. Reaction occurs early during the transfusion.

. Arm pain, chest pain, chills and fever and shock are characteristic; however, there may only be chills and fever.

. Hemolysis is usually intravascular with hemoglobinemia and hemoglobinuria (p. 31).

- Intravascular coagulation and acute renal shutdown are common with severe hemolytic reactions.

Leukoagglutinin Reactions

Such reactions, due to the presence (usually in the recipient) of white cell antibodies, are common, especially in multiply transfused patients, and usually cause chills and fever occurring classically late in transfusion. Such reactions are not usually dangerous and are prevented by using white cell-poor blood components (p. 112) in those patients with a prior history of such reactions.

Approach to "Chills and Fever" Reactions

The house officer's dilemma when faced with a "chills and fever" transfusion reaction involves the difficulty in ruling out the presence of a hemolytic reaction. The following procedure is recommended when faced with a patient experiencing chills and fever while receiving a transfusion.

1. Discontinue the transfusion.

2. Double check the patient's and the blood unit's identification.

3. Obtain a urine and plasma specimen to check for color (red or brown) indicative of hemoglobin or methemoglobin.

4. Return the unit and post-transfusion cross match specimen (and urine sample) to the blood bank.

5. Begin treatment for a presumed hemolytic transfusion reaction if:

    a. The urine/plasma color suggests hemoglobin. (Hemoccult testing of the urine may help, but remember that the test is very sensitive to the presence of any red cells. Serum and plasma samples are almost always contaminated with red cells.)

    b. The patient manifests any of the other symptoms/signs suggestive of a hemolytic transfusion reaction (Table 12.1).

    c. Blood bank re-cross matching indicates an incompatibility.

Most chills and fever reactions are due to leukoagglutinins. It may not be unreasonable to continue the transfusion in the following situations:

1. An identification check reveals the correct unit is hanging, and the patient is known to have had frequent febrile reactions with transfusions, and

2. The reaction is mild and occurring toward the end of the transfusion, and

3. The patient's transfusion history is well known to his physician, and

4. The plasma and urine reveal no evidence of hemoglobin.

However, one must be extremely careful and should err on the side of overreacting to minor transfusion signs and symptoms.

Treatment of a Suspected Hemolytic Reaction

1. Draw bloods for a coagulation screen (DIC is common), baseline renal function tests and electrolytes and for the blood bank for re-cross matching purposes (the patient will probably need further transfusion).

2. Give mannitol in an attempt to establish an osmotic diuresis.

3. Be prepared to provide blood volume expansion to treat shock.

Volume Overload Reactions

Such reactions still remain the most common serious hazard of transfusion. Be careful in the elderly patient or the patient with a history of congestive heart failure, especially if the anemia has developed slowly.

REFERENCE

Mollison PL: Blood Transfusion in Clinical Medicine. Oxford, Blackwell, 1979.

Chapter 13

Polycythemia

One should consider a diagnosis of polycythemia (increased total red blood cell volume) in a man with a persistent hematocrit greater than 55% and in a woman with a persistent hematocrit greater than 50%. Remember decreased plasma volume may result in an elevated hematocrit as well.

It is important to diagnose the presence of polycythemia primarily because of the therapeutic implications of a diagnosis of <u>primary polycythemia</u> (polycythemia vera). Table 13.1 contrasts primary and secondary polycythemia.

<u>Table 13.1</u>
<u>Comparison of Primary and Secondary Polycythemia</u>

	Polycythemia Vera	Secondary Polycythemia
RBC mass	↑	↑
WBCs	Usually ↑	Normal
Basophils	Usually ↑	Normal
Platelets	Usually ↑	Normal
Platelet morphology	Usually abnormal	Normal
Spleen size	Usually ↑	Normal
Leukocyte alkaline phosphatase	Usually ↑	Normal
Serum B12	Usually ↑	Normal
Itching	Common	Uncommon

APPROACH TO WORKUP OF AN ELEVATED HCT

The following is offered as a logical stepwise approach to the diagnosis and evaluation of an elevated Hct:

1. Are any clinical features suggestive of polycythemia vera present?

- Itching

- History of arterial thrombosis

- Splenomegaly

- Elevated WBC

- Basophilia

- Elevated Platelet count

- Abnormal platelet morphology on smear

2.   If any of the above are present (particularly splenomegaly, thrombo-cytosis or leukocytosis), this suggests a diagnosis of polycythemia vera and the physician should complete the workup:

- RBC mass

- Leukocyte alkaline phosphatase

- Vitamin B12 level

A bone marrow examination is not absolutely necessary but may be helpful. It classically reveals marked hypercellularity of all marrow elements and the absence of iron on a marrow iron stain.

3.   If none of the above features is present, polycythemia vera is unlikely. The most likely etiologies are:

a.   Shrunken plasma volume. Acute dehydration without an increase in RBC mass is a common explanation.

b.   Hypoxia. This is by far the most common etiology of secondary polycythemia. Pulmonary function studies and oxygen desaturation on blood gas determination may be diagnostic.

c.   "Gaisbock's syndrome" (stress polycythemia). One commonly sees an elevated hematocrit in middle-aged men who smoke, are plethoric and hypertensive and who have none of the clinical features of polycythemia vera. The RBC mass is usually normal (high normal) and the plasma volume decreased. Many do not consider this a syndrome but just one end of the normal bell-shaped curve. Remember that smoking alone may elevate the hematocrit because of the formation of carboxy-hemoglobin.

4.   If none of the above explanations fit and if the hematocrit is persistently elevated, the physician should document the presence of polycythemia with an RBC mass determination. If elevated,

investigation for one of the less common causes of polycythemia should be undertaken:

a. Erythropoietin producing tumors:

Renal cysts are most common with hypernephroma and hepatomas the next most common etiologies.

b. Methemoglobin, sulfhemoglobin (nitrates in well water, congenital methemoglobinemia, rare).

c. Hemoglobinopathy (e.g., Hgb Chesapeake). The oxygen dissociation curve is shifted to the left with resulting tissue ischemia and secondary increase in the erythropoietin (rare).

d. Cyanotic heart disease.

e. Carboxyhemoglobin. As mentioned above, smoking may raise the hematocrit several percentage points.

TREATMENT

Secondary Polycythemia

For the most part no specific treatment is directed toward the polycythemia. Phlebotomy is rarely indicated in severe pulmonary hypoxemia or congenital heart disease. Treatment should be directed at the underlying etiology: stopping smoking, improving pulmonary function, eliminating nitrate exposure, treatment of the underlying tumor or cysts, etc.

Polycythemia Vera

. Phlebotomy

The mainstay of treatment is phlebotomy to a normal RBC mass. It is important to phlebotomize to iron deficiency (low MCV) in order to eliminate an ongoing need for frequent phlebotomy. For the most part the objective is to keep the hematocrit around 45% and the MCV in the iron-deficient range. It is useful to check the RBC mass periodically to make sure it is normal, as thrombotic complications of this disease correlate better with the RBC mass than the Hct. The itching experienced by many of these patients may not be controlled by phlebotomy. It is useful to avoid hot baths if possible. Antihistamines help little.

. Alkylating Agents or ^{32}p

The use of such agents is controversial. A recent national study suggests there is a significant increase in the risk of developing acute leukemia when they are used. However, there is some further decrease in the incidence of thrombotic events when they are combined with phlebotomy as compared with the use of phlebotomy alone. Survival appears to be unaffected. They should be considered in the patient with a very high platelet count who experiences an arterial thrombotic event in the face of adequate phlebotomy therapy.

• Surgery

It is clear that surgery in the uncontrolled polycythemia vera patient is quite hazardous (bleeding and thrombotic complications). The RBC mass should be normalized before any major surgical procedure.

REFERENCES

Balurzak SP, Bromberg PA: Secondary polycythemia. Semin Hematol 12:353, 1975.

Berk PD, et al: Increased incidence of acute leukemia in polycythemia vera associated with chlorambusil therapy. N Engl J Med 304:441-337, 1982.

Berlin NI: Diagnosis and classification of the polycythemias. Semin Hematol 12:339, 1975.

Silverstein, MN: The evolution into and the treatment of late stage polycythemia vera. Semin Hematol 13:79, 1976.

Wasserman LR, Gilbert HS: Surgery in polycythemia vera. N Engl J Med 269:1226, 1963.

Weinred NJ, Shih CF: Spurious polycythemia. Semin Hematol 12:397, 1975.

Chapter 14

White Cells:
Quantitative Abnormalities

When confronted with an abnormal WBC, the physician should first calculate the absolute count of each of the peripheral blood white cell forms in order to determine precisely the abnormality which needs to be explained.

Calculation of Absolute Counts

Absolute count = total WBC x differential % of individual cell types. This should be determined for:

• Granulocytes

Neutrophils
Eosinophils
Basophils

• Lymphocytes

• Monocytes

Table 14.1
Normal Absolute Counts (Adults)

Neutrophils	1,800-8,000/μl
Eosinophils	0- 600/μl
Basophils	0- 200/μl
Lymphocytes	1,000-5,000/μl
Monocytes	0- 800/μl

The accuracy of absolute counts determined by this method is poor when cells represent fewer than 5-10% of all the white cells (e.g., eosinophils, basophils), and special direct counting techniques are needed if accuracy is important (e.g., eosinophil counts in asthma).

Neutrophilia

Definition

Absolute neutrophil count greater than 8,000 per ml.

Mechanism

Most neutrophilias are due to increased marrow proliferation. However, redistribution of cells among the various body neutrophil pools is the explanation for some neutrophilias. For example:

1. Acute stress (exercise, endogenous or exogenous steroids, epinephrine, sepsis) causes a shift of cells out of the marrow into the peripheral blood and a redistribution of cells from the marginal pool (cells sequestered in the micro-circulation and along blood vessel walls which are not counted by the WBC) to the counted peripheral circulating pool.

2. Chronic steroid administration causes a decreased exodus of peripheral neutrophils to the tissues and a neutrophilia.

Table 14.2
Common Causes of Neutrophilia

Most causes of acute and chronic inflammation
Stress (emotional and physical)
Infections
Tumors
Drugs (steroids, epinephrine, lithium)
Splenectomy
Hemorrhage
Hemolytic anemia
Convulsions
Myeloproliferative disorders

Neutrophilic Leukemoid Reactions

"Leukemoid" refers to a persistent high WBC (usually neutrophilia) suggestive of leukemia. Counts may reach 50,000-100,000 cells per μl, and occasionally counts greater than 100,000 per μl are seen. Infection, inflammation and tumors are the usual causes. The type of leukemia usually suggested by a neutrophilic leukemoid reaction is chronic granulocytic leukemia (CGL).

Table 14.3
Comparison of CGL and Leukemoid Reaction

	Leukemoid Reaction	CGL
Total Count	Usually < 100,000/μl	May be > 300,000/μl
Degree of left shift	Minimal	Large (blasts may be seen)
Basophils	Normal	Increased
Splenomegaly	Usually absent	Usually present
Leukocyte alkaline phosphate staining	Increased	Decreased or absent

Neutrophil Morphology in Infection

The individual neutrophil morphology on a peripheral smear in patients with a bacterial infection may be quite characteristic (must be a fingerstick preparation as anticoagulant may spuriously cause similar changes):

1. Toxic granulations (coarse cytoplasmic granules). This is a nonspecific finding and may be seen in inflammation, cancer and other conditions as well.

2. Döhle bodies (sky blue cytoplasmic inclusions). Sometimes the whole cytoplasm takes on a muddy, light blue color. More specific than toxic granulations but not pathognomonic of infection.

3. Cytoplasmic vacuoles (single or multiple and may be seen in only a small percentage of the cells). Reasonably specific for a bacterial infection. Anticoagulant will cause vacuoles, so the preparation must be a fingerstick. Note that monocytes may have vacuoles normally, even on a fingerstick.

Eosinophilia

Definition

Absolute eosinophil count greater than 600 per μl. Note that direct counting methods are more accurate when the eosinophil percentage is less than 5-10%.

Table 14.4
Common Causes of Eosinophilia

Parasites
Allergic reactions (including drugs)
Dermatitis
Hodgkin's disease
Myeloproliferative disease
Adrenal insufficiency
Chronic renal disease
Radiotherapy
Drugs
Collagen vascular disease

In general, diagnostic evaluation of mild eosinophilia is frequently not fruitful, but total eosinophil counts greater than 4,000 per µl can usually be explained.

Massive eosinophilia may be seen in a very rare group of disorders called the hypereosinophilic syndromes.

Basophilia

Definition

Basophils are found easily on the peripheral smear and represent considerably more than 2-3% of the differential.

Table 14.5
Common Causes of Basophilia

Hypersensitivity reactions
Myeloproliferative disorders

    Polycythemia vera
    Agnogenic myeloid metaplasia
    Primary thrombocythemia
    CGL

Postsplenectomy
Inflammatory states

The presence of increased numbers of basophils may be particularly helpful as a diagnostic clue of the presence of a myeloproliferative disorder.

Monocytosis

Definition

An absolute monocyte count greater than 800 per μl in an adult.

Table 14.6
Common Causes of Monocytosis

Almost any inflammatory condition
Malignancy
SBE
Tuberculosis
Other infections
Collagen vascular disease
Myeloproliferative syndromes
Hodgkin's disease
Leukemias
Preleukemic syndrome
Neutropenia
During recovery from agranulocytosis

The differential diagnosis of monocytosis is so extensive that its presence is usually not helpful in approaching the differential diagnosis of a clinical problem.

Lymphocytosis

Definition

An absolute lymphocyte count greater than 5,000 per μl.

Table 14.7
Common Causes

Normal morphology

Pertussis
Acute infectious lymphocytosis
Chronic lymphocytic leukemia
Waldenstrom's macroglobulinemia (sometimes normal
  morphology)
Thyrotoxicosis

(continued on following page)

Table 14.7 Cont'd)

Atypical lymphocytes (nonmalignant)

Infectious mononucleosis
Cytomegalovirus infection
Viral Hepatitis
Other viral illnesses
Toxoplasmosis
Typhoid fever
Allergic reactions (drugs, etc.)

Abnormal morphology (malignant)

Lymphosarcoma cell leukemia
Acute lymphatic leukemia
Mycosis fungoides, Sezary syndrome

The experienced observer can usually distinguish between the morphology of the pleomorphic atypical lymphocytes seen in benign (usually viral or allergic) conditions and the abnormal lymphocytes seen in malignant lymphoproliferative diseases. In benign conditions the bone marrow usually does not show a marked lymphocytosis.

Neutropenia

Definition

An absolute neutrophil count in an adult of less than 1,800 per μl. It should be noted that 1,500 per μl is the lower range of normal in some studies and that 2% of a normal population will have counts less than these lower limit values. The black population in the United States has a lower normal neutrophil limit than the Caucasian population.

Defining the Mechanism

Persistent neutropenia, even of a mild degree, not obviously explained by an acute event (such as a viral infection) must be evaluated and a specific etiology defined if possible.

Routine Data Base

.   CBC

.   Bone marrow aspiration and biopsy

.   Evaluation of spleen size (PE, spleen scan)

The above data should help to place the neutropenia into one of the following categories as to mechanism:

1.   Decreased bone marrow proliferation

2.   Ineffective bone marrow production

3.   Decreased neutrophil survival

4.   Redistribution neutropenia (margination)

1. Decreased Bone Marrow Proliferation

Common Etiologies

Aplastic anemia
Marrow infiltration (myelophthisis)
Acute agranulocytosis
Drug-induced neutropenia or aplasia

The bone marrow reveals a decrease in granulocyte precursors and may indicate a specific etiology in the case of marrow infiltrative diseases such as leukemia, metastatic cancer, etc. A drug-induced etiology is most common.

Drug-induced Hypoproliferative Neutropenia

a.   Universal, Dose Related

Most of the chemotherapeutic agents used in oncology cause a dose-related neutropenia (and usually thrombocytopenia) in everyone. Other agents, not usually thought of as marrow suppressive, will cause neutropenia in everyone if used in large enough doses. These include:

   .   Chloramphenicol

   .   Ethanol

   .   Rifampin

b.   Idiosyncratic, Dose Related

These drugs cause neutropenia only in some individuals. Usually the drug has to be taken in large doses for a period of time (at least 2 weeks) prior to the onset of neutropenia. Unrecognized host factors are a prerequisite. The best studied drug in this category is chlorpromazine, which is known to inhibit DNA synthesis. Neutropenia usually develops during the first 3 months of therapy or not at all. Frequently, the neutropenia is mild (may be severe), and the white count rapidly reverts to normal after discontinuation of the drug. Other agents (less well studied) which may fall in this category of drug-induced neutropenia include:

- Antithyroid agents

- Other phenothiazines

- Imipramine

- Antibiotics

> Chloramphenicol
> Sulfonamides
> Carbenicillin
> Isoniazid

- Antihistamines (e.g., pyribenzamine)

- Phenylbutazone

- Penicillamine

c. <u>Hypersensitivity Reactions</u>

Some drug-induced neutropenias appear to be allergic, hypersensitivity reactions, suggesting an antibody mechanism (for
the most part not well proven). Such reactions do not appear
to be dose related and are frequently accompanied by eosinophilia.
Drugs reputed to give this type of reaction include:

- Sulfonamides

- Ampicillin

- Chloramphenicol

- Penicillin

- Phenylbutazone

- Quinidine

- Procainamide

- Diuretics (thiazides, ethacrynic acid)

<u>Acute Agranulocytosis</u>

Severe isolated drug-induced production neutropenia with
an absolute neutrophil count less than 200 is called <u>acute agranulo-
cytosis</u>. It is seen with idiosyncratic and hypersensitivity
reactions primarily and is a life-threatening illness (20% mortality). Recovery usually occurs within 2 weeks after discontinuing

the drug. Treatment involves recognition, discontinuation of all possible offending drugs, hospitalization and broad-spectrum antibiotic coverage for any fever.

Aplastic Anemia

Acute agranulocytosis is a short self-limited illness with complete recovery if the patient survives the short neutropenia period. In contrast, aplastic anemia, which may occur as a hypersensitivity reaction to certain drugs, is usually chronic and frequently fatal. Bone marrow transplantation has become the procedure of choice for the young patient with severe aplasia and the availability of a HLA identical sibling. Androgens may occasionally be useful in the patient with mild aplasia.

d. Chronic Neutropenia or Pancytopenia with Decreased Marrow Precursors.

In vitro bone marrow culture techniques may be useful to distinguish cases due to nonimmune stem cell damage from those due to immunologic stem cell suppression. Anecdotal responses in this latter group have been reported with steroids, antilymphocyte globulin, splenectomy, plasmaphoresis, etc.

2. Ineffective Bone Marrow Production

Common Etiologies

Megaloblastic anemia

Folate deficiency
B12 deficiency
Drugs which interfere with folate metabolism
(methotrexate, hydroxyurea, cytosine arabinoside,
pyrimethamine, diphenylhydantoin)

Preleukemia

The bone marrow is cellular but discloses qualitative abnormalities usually of all cell lines. There is intramarrow cell death and frequently peripheral cytopenia. In B12 and folic acid deficiency the peripheral neutropenia rapidly corrects with appropriate vitamin treatment.

3. Decreased Neutrophil Survival

Some patients with autoimmune disease such as SLE and Felty's syndrome have chronic neutropenia secondary to antineutrophil antibodies. Some drug-induced neutropenias may also be secondary to autoantibodies to peripheral neutrophils. In vitro detection of antineutrophil antibodies is difficult, the multiple tests suffering from problems of specificity. The bone marrow, in such patients, is cellular but usually reveals only early precursors ("maturation arrest" picture), The more mature cells being released to the peripheral circulation early.

Such a mechanism for leukopenia, even when severe, is usually less dangerous and life threatening than production neutropenias of the same degree. Remember:

. The peripheral pool of granulocytes is quite small in comparison to the marrow pools.

. Cells pass through the peripheral pool rapidly (in a few hours) on their way to the tissues.

. A neutrophil count, therefore, gives little information pertinent to the important issue – the number of cells being delivered to the tissues.

. Worry more about severe neutropenia with a hypoplastic bone marrow (agranulocytosis, aplastic anemia).

. Worry less about severe neutropenia with a hypercellular bone marrow.

4. Redistribution Neutropenia

Normally the peripheral blood granulocytes are distributed about equally between a "circulating pool" of cells measured by the peripheral neutrophil count and a "marginal pool" of cells distributed along vessel walls, in the microcirculation and in the spleen (not counted by a neutrophil count). Cells may shift from the circulating pool to the marginal pool, giving a false impression of neutropenia in the following circumstances:

. Hypersplenism

. Overwhelming bacterial sepsis

. Viremia

Tissue delivery is frequently adequate even though the peripheral neutrophil count suggests otherwise. Bone Marrow granulocyte precursors are adequate or increased.

Lymphopenia

Definition

An absolute lymphocyte count of less than 1,000 per μl is usually considered abnormal, although in one series 6% of a normal population had counts less than 1,000 per μl. Lymphocytopenia has little diagnostic significance and is frequently unexplained. Conditions known to be associated include:

- Congenital immunologic deficiency syndromes
- Malignancy
- Hodgkin's disease
- Chemotherapy
- Radiotherapy
- Collagen vascular 'disease
- Inflammation
- Corticosteroid excess
- Uremia
- Acute alcoholism

REFERENCES

Cassileth PA: Monocytosis. In Williams WJ, et al: Hematology ed 2,New York, McGraw-Hill, 1977, p 974.

Finch SC: Granulocytopenia. In Williams WJ, et al: Hematology, ed 2, New York, McGraw-Hill, 1977, p 717.

Finch SC: Granulocytosis. In Williams WJ, et al: Hematology, ed 2, New York, McGraw-Hill, 1977, p 746.

Logue GL, Shimms DS: Autoimmune granulocytopenia. In Creger WP et al: Annual Review of Medicine, Vol 31, Palo Alto, 1980, p 191.

Pisciotta AV: Drug-induced leukopenia and aplastic anemia. Clin Pharmacol Ther 12:13, 1971.

Zacharski LR, Elveback LR, Linman JW: Leukocyte counts in healthy adults. Am J Clin Pathol 56:148, 1971.

Zacharski LR, Linman JW: Lymphocytopenia: its causes and significance. Mayo Clin Proc 46:168, 1971.

Chapter 15

Infectious Mononucleosis

Infectious mononucleosis is an acute febrile illness seen primarily in teenagers and young adults; it is classically associated with pharyngitis, lymphadenopathy, splenomegaly and marked atypical lymphocytosis. Characteristic signs and symptoms are listed in the table below.

Table 15.1
Signs and Symptoms of Infectious Mononucleosis

Common Symptoms	Common Signs	
Malaise	Adenopathy	(100%)
Warmth, chilliness	Pharyngitis	(85%)
Sore throat	Fever	(90%)
Myalgia	Splenomegaly	(60%)
Headache	Bradycardia	(40%)
Cough	Periorbital edema	(25%)
Anorexia	Palatal enanthem	(25%)

Less Common Signs and Symptoms

Jaundice	(10%)
Arthralgia	(5%)
Skin rash	(5%)
Diarrhea	(5%)
Photophobia	(5%)

Remember the following:

1. The pharyngitis may be severe and is frequently accompanied by an exudate which is foul smelling, rarely with some degree of respiratory obstruction.

2. Posterior cervical adenopathy is characteristic, but there is usually generalized lymph node enlargement.

3. Ten to 15% of patients have an illness characterized by nonspecific malaise, fever, etc., without pharyngitis.

4. In the very young and the elderly, signs and symptoms are less specific, and pharyngitis is less common.

5. The course may be protracted, with nonspecific symptoms, lymphadenopathy and splenomegaly persisting for weeks. Most patients are significantly improved by 3 weeks.

BASIC LABORATORY FEATURES

White count: Usually elevated (between 10,000 and 20,000 per μl), with maximal counts occurring during the second and third weeks of the clinical illness.

Neutrophil count: An absolute neutropenia is common, and occasionally neutrophil counts less than 500 per μl are seen.

Lymphocytes: There is almost always an absolute lymphocytosis (greater than 5,000 per μl which is maximal during the second week of the clinical illness. Lymphocytes have atypical morphology characterized by pleomorphism.

Hematocrit: Usually normal. Mild hemolysis may occur occasionally, and, rarely, severe Coombs'-positive hemolysis is seen.

Platelet count: A mild thrombocytopenia (usually with counts greater than 100,000 per μl) is not unusual. Severe thrombocytopenia which appears to be immunologically mediated occurs, but it is quite rare.

Liver function tests: Mild liver enzyme abnormalities are common, and up to 50% of patients will show mild hyperbilirubinemia. Enzyme levels essentially never reach the levels seen in viral hepatitis.

Cold agglutinins: Frequently elevated (without hemolysis) due to an antibody directed against the i red cell antigen.

SEROLOGIC TESTS

Heterophil Antibodies

Elevated in 90% of patients, although elevation may not be detected until the third week of clinical illness. Differential absorption studies are necessary to identify the presence of those heterophil antibodies specific for infectious mononucleosis (absorbed by beef red cells but not guinea pig kidney).

Horse Cell Agglutinins (e.g., the "Monospot" test)

The use of horse red cells affords increased specificity over the use of sheep red cells. This is a very good screening test for infectious mononucleosis. Again, maximal positivity of the test occurs during the third week of the clinical illness.

Antibodies to the Epstein-Barr Virus (EBV)

The EBV is the etiologic agent in infectious mononucleosis. A number of serologic assays for specific antibodies to various antigenic components of EBV are currently available. They are primarily helpful in distinguishing EBV positive, heterophile negative infectious mononucleosis from the infectious mononucleosis syndrome due to other etiologic agents (e.g., CMV). They may also be useful in clarifying the etiology in patients with a recurrent infectious mononucleosis syndrome.

. IgM antibody to viral capsid antigen (IgM anti-VCA). Rises early in primary infection with EBV.

. IgG antibody to viral capsid antigen (IgG anti-VCA). Rises slightly later than IgM anti-VCA and remains detectable for life.

. Antibodies to the early antigen (EA) complex of EBV. Two components are recognized, the diffuse (D) and restricted (R). Anti-D antibodies rise early in primary infection and disappear by 2-3 months.

. Antibodies to EB nuclear antigen (EBNA). Anti-EBNA rise very late (months) after primary infection and are detectable for life.

DIFFERENTIAL DIAGNOSIS

Although a number of infections and even malignant conditions may mimic infectious mononucleosis, the following conditions are those most likely to give confusion:

1. Cytomegalovirus infection. Pharyngitis is much less common, as is lymphadenopathy. Probably accounts for the majority of cases of seronegative mononucleosis.

2. Toxoplasmosis. Pharyngitis is less common, but otherwise some cases (a minority) of acquired toxoplasmosis may closely mimic infectious mononucleosis. Diagnosis is usually established by the demonstration of a rising IgM toxoplasmosis titer.

3. Miscellaneous. Bacterial pharyngitis, acute leukemia, infectious hepatitis, other viral illnesses.

COMPLICATIONS

Severe complications are quite rare:

1. **Neurologic.** Includes encephalitis, meningitis, peripheral neuropathy and the Guillain-Barré syndrome. Deaths have been reported, especially with the latter syndrome.

2. Occasional superinfection with bacterial infections has been reported, sometimes in association with agranulocytosis.

3. **Splenic rupture.** A number of deaths from spontaneous splenic rupture have been reported. Diagnosis is easy to miss. Be wary of a history of sudden, brief, sharp abdominal pain.

4. **Other** severe complications (rarely fatal) include myocarditis, hepatic necrosis and airway obstruction.

TREATMENT

There is no specific therapy other than supportive care, treatment of superinfection and surgery for splenic rupture. There are no good data demonstrating that prolonged bed rest is helpful. Steroids are reserved usually for patients with severe pharyngitis and impending airway obstruction and are usually dramatically effective. Avoid antibiotics, especially ampicillin, which has been reported to commonly cause a severe rash in patients with infectious mononucleosis.

REFERENCES

Carter RL, Penman HG, eds: Infectious Mononucleosis. Oxford, Blackwell, 1969.

Evans AS, Niederman JC, McCallul RW: Seroepidemiologic studies of infectious mononucleosis with EB virus. N Engl J Med 279:1121, 1968.

Hoagland RJ: Infectious Mononucleosis. New York, Grune & Stratton, 1969.

Horwitz CA: Practical approach to diagnosis of infectious mononucleosis. Postgrad Med 65:No.6:179, 1979.

Horwitz CA, et al: Heterophil-negative infectious mononucleosis and mononucleosis-like illness. Amer J Med 63:947, 1977.

Index